Copyright © 2009-2011 by Jayme Hunt, Christine Hunt, MadeInBoyd.com, LessofMeHCG.com
All rights reserved.

Published in the United States of America
By Jayme Hunt & Christine Hunt, MadeInBoyd.com, LessofMeHCG.com

First Edition published November 6, 2009

Cover art, jacket design, and images Copyright © 2009-2011, Jayme Hunt & Christine Hunt

No part of this book may be reproduced, stored in a retrieval system, or transmitted in any form or by any means, electronic, mechanical, photocopying, recording, scanning, or otherwise, except as permitted under Section 107 or 108 of the 1976 United States Copyright Act, without the prior written permission of the Author.

The product names used in this book are for identification purposes only. All trademarks and registered trademarks are the property of their respective owners. Other company, product, and service names may be trademarks or service marks of others.

100 Recipes
to keep you on
Phase II
of
HCG

A "Less of Me" Publication by
Christine Hunt
&
Jayme Hunt

Limit of Liability & Disclaimer:

The stories in this book are from personal experience by either Jayme or Christine. Neither of them are health professionals. In preparing this book, the authors put forth their best efforts but make no representation or warranties with respect to the accuracy or completeness of the contents of this book. The authors further disclaim any implied warranties for a particular purpose. The recipes and HCG diet may not be suitable for your particular situation. No warranty may be created or extended by sales representatives or written sales materials. You should consult a professional where appropriate. Neither authors will be liable for loss of profit or other commercial damages including special, incidental, consequential, or other damages.

If you choose to use the information in this book without a health professional's aid and approval, you self prescribe. Neither author assumes responsibility for how you use the information in this book. The authors will not be held responsible for misuse of the product or recommendations. By reading this book, you acknowledge that this information is to be used for entertainment or educational purposes only and does not replace the advice of a health professional.

Legally, the authors must state:
The statements in this book have not been evaluated by the Food & Drug Administration. None of the products listed or mentioned should be used as a substitute for medical advice, nor to diagnose, treat, or cure any illness. The FDA has not approved HCG for weight loss and there is no substantial evidence that HCG is effective in the treatment of obesity.

Note:
For the record, the authors disagree with the FDA, based on their personal experiences with the HCG Protocol and looking at their images before and after following the protocol.

Dedication

For 9 year old Daphne, who tells us our butts are smaller.
For 8 year old Devon, who tells us he loves us even if we are fat.
And for all the readers of our blog, LessofMeHCG.com,
who encouraged us to create this cookbook.

~Christine & Jayme

A Note from the Authors

Ultimately, the success following a protocol like HCG comes from within. YOU have control of your world and your body. We left this page black and white because that's what following the protocol is about.

You do it or you don't.

If you do it, you'll be rewarded with contrasting images of yourself as obvious as black and white.

And you'll be so happy with yourself.

Here's to Less of Me and You!

~Christine & Jayme

Index

Introductions
Christine..5
Jayme..6

Staple Sauces
Ketchup...9
Worcester Sauce...9
Garlic Butter..9
Teriyaki..10
BBQ...10
Marinara..10

Beef
Balsamic Roast Beef..14
Cabbage Rolls & Kraut....................................15
Coffee Roast Beef...16
Garlic Basil Roast Beef....................................17
Garlic Curry Beef Soup...................................18
Home on The Range Steak............................19
Japanese Steak..20
Orange BBQ Steak..22
Safeggheti...23
Zucchini Basil Soup..24
Zucchini Meatloaf..25

Beverages
Cocoa..28
   White Dark
   Raspberry
   Chocolate Strawberry Crème
   Orange
   Peppermint
Coffee..29
   Mocha Frappè
   French Vanilla
   Raspberry Mocha
   Caramel
   Caramel Mocha Frappè
   Vanilla Toffee
Tea..30
   Fairy Rooibus
   Vanilla Rooibus Crème
   Chocolate Mint
   Vanilla Mint
   Vanilla Orange Rooibus
Savory...31
   Vegetable
   Tomato Sipper
   Basil

Buffalo
Buffalo Celery Soup..34
Buffalo Chili..35
Buffalo Chips...36
Buffalo Meatballs & Sour Kraut....................37
Buffaloaf..38
Running with the Buffalo Soup....................39
Tomato Basil Soup...40

Chicken
Autumn Bliss Soup...43
Asian Garlic..44
Balsamic Mustard...45
Bar the Barley Soup...46
Chicken Celery Aspic.......................................47
Chicken Sausage..48
Tomato Soup-erior...49
Chili Tomato Chicken......................................50
Cola Chicken..51
Cucumber Chicken Salad...............................54
Herb Marinated Chicken................................55

Lazy Sunday Chicken..........................56
Non Ton Soup.....................................57
Orange Chicken Stirfry.......................58
Orange Ginger Chicken......................59
Raspberry Mustard Chicken...............60
Savory Chicken & Apples...................61
Sott'er celo de Roma..........................63
Up Town Chicken Soup......................65

Fish
Broccoli Fish Soup..............................67
Buttery Orange Roughy......................68
Cod Bake..69
Herb the Halibut.................................70
It's a Keeper!......................................71
Orange Roughy Soup.........................72

Lobster
St. Barth Seafood Salad.....................74

Shrimp
Baked Shrimp.....................................76
Dilly Garlic Shrimp..............................77
Honey Citrus Glazed Shrimp..............78
Ran Out of Time Asian Shrimp...........79
Shrimp Cocktail..................................80
Wannabe Sushi..................................81
Zippy Shrimp......................................82

Veggie
Dilled Cabbage...................................14
Apple Celery Soup..............................84
Cole Slaw...85
Liquid Sunshine Soup.........................86
Waldorf Salad & Vinnegrape Dressing.............87

Desert
Apple Chips..89
Sweet Toffee Apple............................90
Baked Apple.......................................91
Orange Crème de Licious..................92
Raspberry Apple.................................93
Tart Toffee Apple................................94
Yogurt...95
    Lemon Christilicious
    Cinnamon
    Lime
    Raspberry Cheesecake
    Strawberry Pudding
    Apple Pudding
    Orange Jaymeus
Raspberry Jello..................................98
Raspberry Sorbet...............................99

Comments
Overview of what we get to eat...........7
Liquid Aminos, a quick study.............11
Not a Happy Camper..........................21
10 Likely Culprits for Stalls................26
Of Habits and Hangups.....................32
It's Never Been This Easy.................41
Eating Out..52
A Funny..66
Apple Day..73
Scale Fairy...75
A Funny This Morning........................83
Raspberry Picking..............................88
Egg Day..100
Final Notes.......................................102
Resources..104
About the Authors............................106

This cookbook has been a challenge.

The HCG diet has been a challenge.

When I first looked at the food item list and the amount of calories allowed per day I thought it would be impossible. But I am nothing, if not a dreamer, and my dream to be thin and healthy over rode my fear of failure. Besides that, I am not one to steer clear of a challenge.

I have been cooking and baking for more than 40 years. I remember learning to make Baking Powder Biscuits in 4-H. The oldest of six children in a single parent household, our family was at or below the poverty level, and our diet suffered because of it. I think between the foods we received through the government program and my family genes I was doomed from the outset to be overweight, which isn't to say I haven't "enjoyed" eating my way there. I had myself convinced after years of yo-yo dieting that I would never diet again. But when I reached 230 pounds on my 5'5" frame my blood pressure skyrocketed, I was facing medication or another diet.

The HCG diet isn't unlike other diets that I had tried. I'd done 500 calorie diets before. It was doable. But before HCG, it was miserable. What I liked about the idea of HCG was there was a time limit, thirty days, no problem. And if I could lose as many pounds in that time, then I was on board. But the best part was that all my reading indicated this would be a permanent weight loss. The promise to re-set my body's ideal weight was tantalizing. What did I have to lose? Thirty days out of my life was little enough to pay.

And so we began. It helps to have a partner and I had a good one. Jayme intends to blog her way through more than 150 pounds of weight loss. Along the way, she shared our creative recipes, and the response was tremendous. I never realized how many people out there don't (or can't) cook. And so the idea of creating this HCG cook book was born.

We hope you enjoy the variety of foods and preparations of the recipes in this book and that it will help you to stick with the program. It isn't hard. In fact, I wasn't hungry and I didn't crave any of the foods I couldn't eat the whole way through my HCG experience. Each recipe is packed with flavor and designed to help you be successful.

Here's to "Less of Me" and YOU!

~Christine

I started following the HCG Protocol in September 2009. My start weight was 332 pounds. During my first round, which is where these recipes all came from, I released 47 pounds. (I don't lose weight – losing things means you want to find them again later!) I've still got another hundred pounds to release, scheduled for 2010, and I'm going to continue following the HCG protocol.

The cool part is this: It just works. That's what I look for when I'm buying just about anything. I want my car to "just work." I want my clothes to "just work" for me. I want my hairspray to "just work." It's silly that all these years, I tried out diets that didn't work long term. And it's even sillier that I followed them when I knew they didn't work. I was just desperate to get rid of the weight and find the confidence in my exterior that I already felt on my interior.

The recipes in this book are ones that I enjoyed while on the protocol. You'll find some recipes to make foods that taste as close to "normal" foods as we could and I'm sure you're going to enjoy them!

I researched HCG for a full year, tracking people who just finished their rounds, to see if the hype of maintaining the new healthy weight was real or not. I was a database administrator for 12 years, so data and tracking things like that comes naturally. What finally pushed me to the point of starting was that all the lines and tracking proved, from normal people, that the hype wasn't hype at all. It was truth. Finally! A method I could use to gain control of my exterior!

There's a lot of embarassing facts and information on my blog and in this book. I choose to share it so that other people – YOU – will know that you can do it, too. I share so that others will find their own starting point and gain control of their exteriors, should they wish it. I decided to track my experiences with a public blog, so I could keep track of what was going on with the protocol and to recall the recipes created, too.

This is actually where this recipe book came from. So many people looked forward to our recipes and encouraged us to design new recipes, that we decided to make a book. How wonderful to be able to help others stay on their HCG path with great recipes so they're not bored or feel like they're missing out. It feels great to help other people, too!

Here's to Less of Me - and You, too! We can do it!

~Jayme

Overview of what we get to eat on HCG

The rules are pretty strict, so here's an overview of them:

- Per meal:
    - 1 vegetable
    - 1 (100g) meat
    - 1 fruit
    - 1 breadstick (they're more like bread pencils, but about twice as long as a pencil)
- Each meal is 250 calories. The meat, breadstick, and fruit calories are then added up, subtracted from the 250 allowed and the rest is consumed in the vegetable.
- Spices (any spice) are allowed in any amounts.
- 1 T milk per day, if desired.
- Juice of 1 lemon per day, if desired.
- 1T Tomato Paste per day, if desired.
- Celtic Sea Salt is the only salt allowed.
- Stevia is the only sweetener allowed.
- The fruit can be postponed from the main meal and used as a snack or desert.
- Tea or coffee can be consumed in any quantities. <-- This one is interesting because I have lots of loose leaf tea that have different flavors like those just below. I thought we might soak something in tea to get the flavor of the tea in it. But, I've NOT done anything like that before so it'll be a stretch of the imagination. :)
    - Georgia Peach Rooibus
    - Vanilla Rooibus
    - Vanilla Honeybush
    - Vanilla St Bourbon Rooibus
    - Cherry Green
    - "Fairy Garden" Rooibus (lavender flavored)

<u>Meats allowed, in 100g quantities (and calories)</u>

Buffalo 100

Chicken Breast 110

Steak 140

Extra Lean Ground Beef 215

Roast Beef 150

Veal 100

Lobster 95

Crab 55

Shrimp 90

Sea Bass 120

Flounder 110

Halibut 100

Sole 120

Orange Roughy 76

Cod 82

Fat Free Cottage Cheese 90

2 c Celery 38

2 c Chard 14

1 c Chicory Greens 41

2 c Cucumbers 29

1 1/2 c Fennel 40

2 c Lettuce 16

1 c Mushrooms 40

2 c Radishes 46

2 c Spinach 13

1 c String Beans 53

1 c Summer Squash 31

1 c Tomatoes 65

1 c Watercress 4

1 c Onions (white, yellow, red) 61

1 c Zucchini 20

Veggies allowed (and calories/serving)

2 c Asparagus 62

2 c Bean Sprouts 46

2 c Beet Greens 46

1 c Broccoli 50

2 c Cabbage 35

1 c Cauliflower 50

Fruits allowed (and calories/serving)

1 medium Apple 80

1/4 Cantaloupe 48

1/2 Grapefruit 40

1 Navel Orange 60

1/2 cup Raspberries 32

6 Strawberries 28

Staple Sauces

Ketchup

1T tomato paste
1pk stevia (approximately 1/2t)
1T apple cider vinegar
1t Worcester sauce
salt and pepper to taste
1T water
Mix all ingredients together. If it's too sweet for your tastes, add more vinegar or water to dilute it down.
Note: This will count as your 1 Tablespoon of Tomato Paste, should you use this!

Worcester Sauce

- 1/2 cup apple cider vinegar
- 2 tablespoons soy sauce
- 2 tablespoons water
- 3 drops toffee stevia
- 1/4 teaspoon ground ginger
- 1/4 teaspoon dry mustard
- 1/4 teaspoon onion powder
- 1/4 teaspoon garlic powder
- 1/8 teaspoon cinnamon
- 1/8 teaspoon pepper

Place all ingredients in a pan and bring to a boil, stirring constantly. Simmer 1 minute with lid on. Cool. Store in the refrigerator in a mason jar.

Garlic Butter
5 calories

1 clove fresh garlic, minced
1t butter buds (5 calories)
3t water
In small dish, mix the butter buds and water together. Add minced garlic and let stand at least 10 minutes so the flavors mingle together.

Staple Sauces

Teriyaki Sauce

1/2c soy sauce
15 drops Stevia
1/2t salt
1 clove minced garlic or 1/2t ginger
Add all ingredients and mix thoroughly. Store in frig.

BBQ Sauce

- 1/4t celery seed
- 1/4t onion powder
- 1/4t garlic powder
- 1/4 cup tomato paste
- 1t ACV (apple cider vinegar - we use Bragg's' ACV)
- 3 drops stevia
- 1 1/4t worcestershire
- 2 drops liquid smoke
- salt & pepper to taste

Add all ingredients and mix thoroughly. Store in frig.
Note: This will count as your 1 Tablespoon of Tomato Paste, should you use this!

Marinara

1T tomato paste
1/8t onion powder
1/8t garlic powder
1/8t italian seasoning
1/8t fennel seed
1 drop stevia
Add all ingredients and mix thoroughly. Store in frig.
Note: This will count as your 1 Tablespoon of Tomato Paste, should you use this!

Amino Acids, a quick overview

I've been getting lots of emails wondering just what good amino acids are and why I use them in my cooking so often. I'll certainly be emailing all those people personally, but I also wanted to address it here on my blog-turned-recipe-book.

Proteins all contain amino acids. Most contain about 9 of the essential amino acids, but there are a full 20 that are essential to the body. Without those 20 aminos, the body starts breaking down lean tissue and muscle. In fact, if you read Nutrition Information's site about aminos , it gets down right scary(http://www.nutritioninformation.us/protein.htm):

> **What happens if an essential amino acid is missing from the body? Well, in the beginning the body will break down lean tissue in order to compensate. Eventually, however, the muscles will begin to waste away. While protein deficiencies are rare in the United States, they are more common in countries with poor diets. In addition to muscle wasting, other signs of protein deficiency include mental impairment in children, edema, anemia, decreased immunity, and metabolic abnormalities.**

Image credit: www.bragg.com

Bragg's Liquid Amino Acids are made from non-GMO soybeans. This is important to me because I figure that our Creator made things just the way we're supposed to be ingesting them. I'm not fond of eating things that have been tampered with because we humans "think" we can out do what's already done in nature. I think that's a terrible folly.

Bragg's FAQ (http://www.bragg.com/products/laFAQ.html) about their amino acids also share with us some further information about aminos and their purpose in our bodies:

> **Amino Acids are the building blocks of all our organs and tissues. They are also the building blocks from which different food proteins are constructed. When we eat a protein food, such as meat or soybeans, the natural hydrochloric acid in the stomach digests the protein, releasing the Amino Acids. They are the link between the food we eat and assimilation for our body tissue. Lack of adequate Amino Acids may make it impossible for the vitamins and minerals to perform their specific duties.**

Myself, I took amino acid pills to alleviate the need for acid reflux medicines before starting this Protocol. If heartburn showed up, I'd pop two amino acid powder pills (it has these two amino acids in it: Arginine and Carnitine) and it would be gone inside of 15 minutes. I also used them to help balance digestive issues when I was detoxing. My Mom uses L-Lysine amino acids to ensure there are no outbreaks of cold sores.

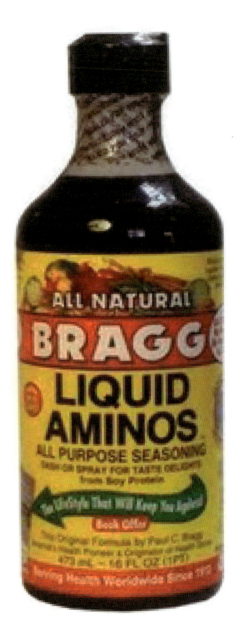

Image credit: www.bragg.com

Bragg's Liquid Amino Acids contains these 16 amino acids in it:

1. Alanine
2. Arginine
3. Aspartic Acid
4. Glutamic Acid
5. Glycine
6. Histidine
7. Isoleucine
8. Leucine
9. Methionine
10. Phenylalanine
11. Proline
12. Serine
13. Threonine
14. Tyrosine
15. Valine
16. Lysine

With the great importance of getting Amino Acids in our bodies, I find that I use it in my cooking quite often. It shouldn't completely take the place of a good quality celtic sea salt, as that has it's own benefits. But, in my opinion, Bragg's should definitely be a part of our every day diet. I think. :)

As of the printing of this book, you can get a free sample of Bragg's Liquid Amino Acids by visiting their sampling section of their website (http://bragg.com), too!

It's easy to cook with, too. It tastes like soy sauce, but not quite as salty. I use it in place of salt, when I want an Asian flavor to my dish, and when I'm dry frying meats.

Tonight, it's time for something a little heavier than normal. Chicken and fishies are nice most of the time, but they leave me feeling "empty." In the summer, I'm a fruit and veggie person - but as it cools off, I want RED MEAT. Roast, steak, hamburger... (<--Read: Dead cow, ready to consume.) It's kind of morbid, I agree, but it is what it is.

I also wanted something different from the roast recipe I came up with already. Something a little more tangy, cooked slower, so the roast would be tender.

Balsamic Roast Beef
150 calories

100g roast beef (150 calories)
sprig of fresh basil
2 cloves garlic, cut into slices
2t Braggs' Liquid Aminos
2T Balsamic Vinegar
pinch nutmeg
salt and pepper to taste

Marinate roast in Braggs' and Balsamic for two hours in the frig. Then, in 8" square of foil, center roast and add pinch nutmeg, salt, pepper, garlic, and basil. Cover and close tightly in the foil, then pop in toaster oven (or conventional oven) at 300* for at least an hour. Serve with your choice of veggie! Seriously yummy.

I wanted to pair this up with a veggie that was low in calories. The fishies are, on average, 50 calories less than beef. That translates to a whole cup less of some sort of veggie. So, I chose cabbage. You get the sharesies on how I steamed it up below:

Dilled Cabbage

Allowed amount of cabbage
3t dill seed
3t salt

Add dill seed and salt to the water. Steam the cabbage up and add a little Braggs' Liquid Aminos to taste and serve up.

Tonight's supper was a real treat, I'll tell you what! It was cabbage several different ways... I baked it, pickled it, and wrapped it. It's lots of steps, but completely worth it in the end. I promise!

Cabbage Rolls & Kraut
250 calories

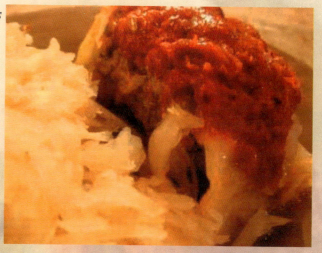

100g hamburger (215 calories)
2 cloves garlic, minced
1t basil
1/2t onion powder
shake of salt and pepper
cabbage leaves (whole leaves from 1/2 the cabbage)
1T tomato paste
1/2t garlic powder
1/2t onion powder
10 fennel seeds
2 drops stevia
1T water
1 1/2c sour kraut (35 calories)
1/2c thinly sliced cabbage

Mix hamburger, minced garlic, basil, 1/2t onion powder, salt and pepper together in small bowl. Set aside. In separate bowl, mix sauce together by adding tomato paste, garlic powder, 1/2t onion powder, fennel seeds, stevia, and water. Stir sauce together and set aside.

Remove a leaf from 1/2 a head of cabbage, trying to leave it in tact as much as possible. Cut out the rib (the hard part in the center of the leaf), then put leaf in a pot of hot water. When leaf is wilted and pliable, remove and run under cold water. Don't dry the leaf off. Place leaf in center of 8" foil and lay it flat. Form a ball of the hamburger mix and wrap the cabbage leaf around the hamburger, tucking the edges under so the meat is completely covered. Top the cabbage/meat with the tomato sauce mixture and fold the foil closed in a pocket. Place in oven at 350* for 50 minutes or until meat is done.

In 8x10 pan, lay thinly sliced cabbage on the bottom. Cover this with sour kraut completely and place in oven at 300* for 30 minutes.

Remove both from oven and place on your dish then enjoy!

Like I said, it's a lot more steps, but the dish is worth it in the end and it's really not that hard. Really, really.

Tonight, for dinner, I had an exceptional meal. No one else uses coffee this way, that I can tell, while on the VLCD. This particular recipe calls for using coffee as a marinade. Coffee lends a deep, strong base to the beef and LOTS of flavor as well as beautiful color. If you have a really good cut of meat, this would be the one recipe I'd recommend for it...

Coffee Roast Beef

150 calories

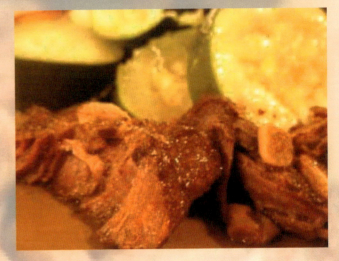

1/2t onion powder
1/4t chili powder
1/4t liquid smoke
1/4t salt
Shake of pepper
2 garlic cloves, sliced
100g roast beef (150 calories)
1 pot of coffee (espresso is best)

In bowl, add onion powder, chili powder, liquid smoke, salt, pepper, cloves. Press meat into spice mixture so it's completely covered (like a rub). Let it sit there while you make a really good strong pot of coffee. Put everything into a bowl, add meat and cover meat with coffee, then cover all of it with foil. (I used a small cereal bowl that was ok to bake in.) Bake at 300* for 3-4 hours.

Chef's Notes:

- *If you have a really good cut of roast beef, you don't need to pound it. If you have a cheap cut, definitely pound it thin first.*
- *This could be a good crock pot recipe, too!*
- *You can save the broth for another recipe or use it on your veggies.*
- *Horse radish added to this recipe would be exceptional! Make sure to read your labels though, to make sure there's no sugar added. Or use fresh grated.*
- *If you saved your broth for a few days, you could add some hamburger, some onion or celery, and make a realllllllly good soup.*

Tonight, we decided to have roast beef. We know that you're only supposed to eat it three times a week, but we've been very good about sticking with fishies, crustaceans, and chickens. It's time to have some MEAT tonight. :)

I did a few things differently than the last two times we've had it. First, we added a whole clove of fresh garlic to each serving of protein. YUM, all by itself. I also added a sprinkle of cinnamon to our meat just before closing up the foil and tossing it into the toaster oven. Those toaster ovens, by the way, are wonderful. You get the same great seasoned taste out of them, but you don't heat up the whole house. Tonight, that's not such a big deal, as it's a little chilly, but normally over Labor Day weekend, it's roasting hot here in Oregon.

So, with all that garlic, you need to be aware that you will, without a doubt, smell of garlic. Please, choose a day to have this when you won't offend others. The crystal, I've found, doesn't do diddly squat for the kind of body odor that comes out ALL your pores. And toothpaste only goes so far. If you're in the presence of others, you could chew on fennel seeds, anise seeds, or a bit of cinnamon bark! Or, if you're just bold and don't care what others think, like me, then enjoy it to the hilt and add a second clove!

Anyway, I digress. Here's the recipe:

Garlic Basil Roast Beef
150 calories

100g Roast Beef (150 calories)
salt & pepper to taste
1/4 t onion powder
1/4 t cinnamon
1 whole fresh garlic clove, sliced into three large slices
1 sprig fresh basil (or 1 t dried)

In an 8" square of foil, place beef in the center. On both sides of beef, sprinkle salt, pepper, & onion powder. On one side, sprinkle cinnamon, place slices of garlic clove, and top with basil sprig. Close the foil over, making a tight pocket to seal in the juices while the meat cooks, and place in toaster oven (or regular oven - that works, too). Bake at 350* for 40 minutes.

We served this beside fresh green beans, steamed then tossed with balsamic vinegar. Hope you enjoy!

Garlic Curry Beef Soup
201 calories

100g steak (140 calories)
onion, cut into 3/4" squares or so (allowed amount) (1c=61 calories)
1T beef bullion
3 cloves minced garlic
1/2t curry powder
1/4t cinnamon
1/4t pumpkin pie spice
2t Bragg's Liquid Aminos
salt & pepper to taste

In pot, bring 1 or 2 cups water, bullion, steak to the

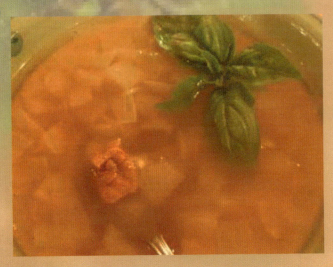

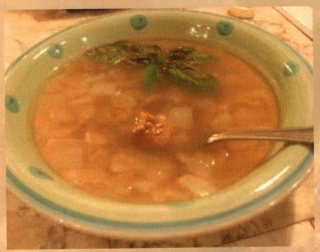

boiling point. While that's heating up, cut up the onion and ready to add it. Just before it starts boiling, remove steak.

Add spices to the broth and stir. Cut up steak into small bite sized pieces and return to broth. Bring to a boil. Reduce heat, cover, and simmer about 45 minutes. Depending on your tastes, this might need a little more salt and pepper, but it generally turns out perfect without needing to add anything to it.

BBQ Sauce

1/4t celery seed
1/4t onion powder
1/4t garlic powder
1/4 cup tomato paste
1t ACV (apple cider vinegar - I use Bragg's ACV)
3 drops stevia
1 1/4t Worcester (see Staple Sauces list)
2 drops liquid smoke
salt & pepper to taste
Add all ingredients and mix thoroughly.

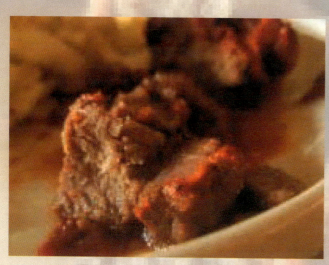

Home on the Range Steak

140 calories

100g steak (140 calories)
BBQ sauce (above)
salt & pepper to taste
In 8" square of foil, center steak, cover with BBQ sauce and place in toaster oven at 350* for 1 hour to make sure the flavors are mingled in with the meat. Fold back the foils and switch your oven to broil and leave for an additional 15 minutes, serve and enjoy!

Yesterday was my planned egg day (6 eggs, by the way, are very satisfying!). It went well! I'm now at my 30 pound milestone!! In any event, I was thinking about this recipe yesterday... Probably because I didn't really have to think about what I was cooking. ::grins::

Japanese Steak

140 calories

100g steak (140 calories)
1T Braggs' Liquid Aminos

1 clove fresh garlic, minced

1/2t grated fresh ginger

1 drop stevia

Mix Braggs', garlic, ginger, and stevia in small bowl. Set aside. Slice steak into strips and add each strip to the marinade bowl. Let stand at least one hour in the frig. Remove from frig and cook in oven at 350* for 10 minutes or until steak is done to your liking.

Not a happy camper

This week, I've not lost a single pound - all week! I thought I did one day, but it turned out that it was just that I weighed in my jammies instead of my clothes. I've never experienced a whole week of feeling like I was going to start *any time now* and then just not.

So, my cycle (grrrrr) has cost me about 14 pounds of weight loss, near as I can calculate.

Today, I experienced my first bad effect of this protocol. Of course, it is during my cycle, so I'm not sure how much I can count it as part of the protocol. I was working working working (we're moving tools from the storage center to the shop so we can get it all set up) and suddenly, without warning, my blood sugar just dropped out the bottom. When that happens, you feel all shaky and like you're going to sick up. However, I didn't have anything in my stomach, so was reasonably sure I wasn't going to do that. I didn't have any meat cooked up yet, so had to wait the 10 minutes it took to cook up some shrimp from frozen. I napped while it was cooking, then crawled over to get the protein. I did NOT CHEAT! It was definitely hard not to, considering I still have cheese (Parmesan and Dubliner's) and some sliced ham for the kids' lunch in the frig and that would normally be what I'd grab first. I'm always careful to keep protein in my system, as I discovered that it's the true key to holding off low blood sugar.

For the record, I'm not diabetic - I've just always been susceptible to low blood sugar when there's not enough protein in my system.

My Mom says I should just push through it, but with the after headache of the low blood sugar and the awful cramps I've had since 2AM, I am not a happy camper.Ugh. Enough of my whining. I've got a new recipe to share with you for a desert next. Stay tuned.

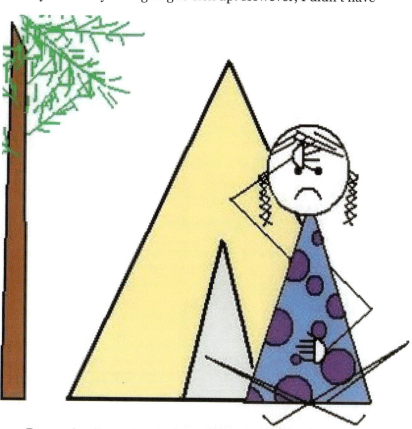

Drawn by Jayme Hunt of Sophisticated Sticks

Orange BBQ Sauce

1/4t celery seed
1T orange juice
1/4t onion powder
1/4t garlic powder
1/4 tomato paste
1t ACV
3 drops stevia
2 drops liquid smoke
salt & pepper to taste
Add all ingredients and mix thoroughly.

Orange Steak
140 calories

100g steak (140 calories)
Orange peel, in one piece if possible!
BBQ sauce (above)
salt & pepper to taste
In 8" square of foil, center orange rind and place steak inside it, cover meat with BBQ sauce and place in toaster oven at 350* for 1 hour to make sure the flavors are mingled in with the meat.

Safegheti

235+ calories

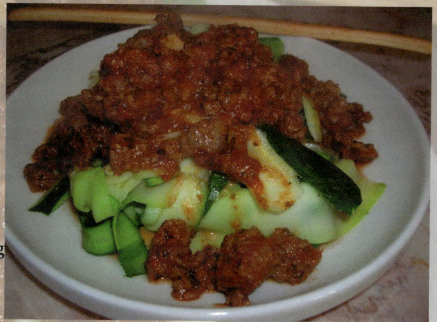

100g ground beef
2 cloves garlic, minced
1T tomato paste
1T onion flakes or 1/2t onion powder
1T Italian Spice
1 1/4t salt (divided)
1 beef bullion cube
1/2c water
allowed amount zucchini

Bring 2 quarts water to a rolling boil. Add 1t salt. On a dry skillet, put meat on to dry fry. Once it's browned, add tomato paste, spices, and 1/2c water. Turn that down and allow to simmer until it's reduced to the thickness you prefer.

Using a potato peeler, slice strips off zucchini so it looks like wide noodles. Lay the zucchini on a cutting board and slice them off. Once the water has come to a rolling boil and your sauce is almost done, put all zucchini in water and blanch it for 1-2 minutes. Empty zucchini into a colander and drain well. Put zucchini on plate, cover with sauce and serve!

Notes: Our Italian Spice mix has marjoram, thyme, rosemary, savory, sage, oregano, & basil.
This would be good over green beans, sauteed onions, mushrooms, or fennel. You could double or triple your recipe and freeze it for a quick meal!

> This particular recipe is one that is *very* close to my all time favorite meal in the whole world. My Mom's Barley Soup. I would rather have that soup than anything available to me, including fettuccine or fondue! And I really love cheese, too.
>
> I never knew how to make the broth and always just begged Mom to make it. It's sort of like her brownies. Where I've never made a pot of it, it's one of those memories from childhood that just shouldn't be messed with as an adult. It's the perfect feel-good food. A whole body full of great feelings gets served up with each spoonful that touches your lips.
>
> There's no pictures of this soup just yet – last time I made it, I could only think about getting that soup into my mouth and getting those great feelings zipping around! I think my family actually liked me better after I ate it.
>
> I couldn't stop smiling.

Zucchini Basil Soup
255 calories

100g hamburger (215 calories)
2c water
1T beef bullion
1t basil
1t onion flakes
2 cloves garlic, minced
1T tomato paste
salt & pepper to taste
2c zucchini (40 calories)

Bring water, bullion, basil, onion, garlic, tomato paste to a boil. Add hamburger and allow to cook. Turn heat down, add zucchini and allow soup to simmer until zucchini is tender. Serve hot and enjoy! You can use any veggie you choose, though!

Zucchini Meatloaf

242 calories

Meatloaf:
100g lean ground beef (215 calories)
1/3 cup grated zucchini (7 calories)
1 grissini breadstick, pulverized (20 calories)
1T milk
1/4t italian seasoning
1/4t garlic powder
1/4t onion powder
a sprinkle of celery seeds

The meal we made last night makes me wish we could have beef every night. We used everything except our fruit in it, including the milk and some tomato paste. And it tasted "normal."

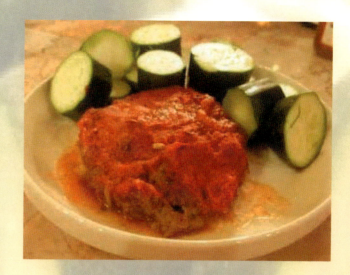

Sauce:
1T tomato paste
1/8t onion powder
1/8t garlic powder
1/8t italian seasoning
1/8t fennel seed
1 drop stevia

Mix meat ingredients together and pat into a patty. Place in center of 8" foil and set aside. Combine sauce ingredients together in bowl and spread on top of patty. Make foil into pocket and cook meatloaf 45 minutes at 350* (toaster ovens work good for this if you don't want to heat the whole house). Uncover meatloaf and broil patty 10 minutes. Then serve it HOT HOT HOT!
Serious NUMMY!! Hope you enjoy it!

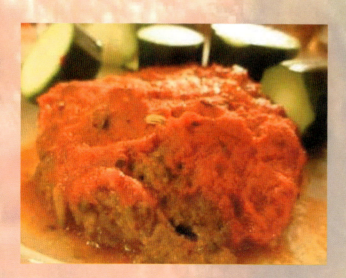

10 Likely Culprits for Stalls

Before I get into the what may be going on part of this, I just wanted to make sure that we're all on the same page about the difference between a plateau and a stall. A plateau should be at least four days. Your first step should be the suggested apple day to see if it shakes things up. If the apple day doesn't work and you find yourself doing everything you're supposed to be doing and your weight is just not moving for five days or more, THEN you are experiencing a stall.

You have to look at the amount of inches you're losing as well as just the weight. I, personally, wasn't happy doing that. Inches is inches, but pounds is pounds. :)

So what to do if you're in a stall? Well, I was in one for 13 days. I went through all these things and finally, when I tried something that's not strictly "on" the protocol, I broke it. I did an egg day, found as a suggestion on a forum I frequent. So, here's my list, albeit long list, of what to look at if you find yourself in this discouraging place.

1. Your body may be just detoxing - try out a long soak in a bath with 2-4 cups of epsom salts. It'll draw out the toxins and you get a great excuse to soak that way.
2. Also, you could increase your water intake, so your body can flush out the fats. You should use your weight, but in ounces (so I'm 300#, I'd use 300 oz for this calculation), then take half of that and that's how much water you should be drinking every day. (I should be drinking 300 oz/2= 150 oz every day.)
3. Do you mix your veggies? If you do, stop.
4. Are you making sure that you've got different meats, veggies, and fruits for lunch than for dinner?
5. Are you taking multivitamins? If you are, there may be hidden sugars in there... It's used for fillers, too.
6. Meat. If you're using just the red meats and skipping the white ones (fish/chicken), your body may just be on red meat overload. Try different meats than you have already.

7. Are you getting enough calories - all 500 - or are you skimping in the hopes of losing more? If you skimp on the calories, you risk your body going into starvation mode and it'll hang onto every calorie it can!

8. Are you allergic to something you're eating/putting on your body? I'm allergic to SLS (sodium laureth sulfate) in the shampoos and ran into some trouble losing because of that. Once I found products that didn't have SLS in it, I started losing again.

9. Not enough sleep! Sleep is when your body repairs itself and makes the large adjustments to the sudden loss of brown fat loss that we're all releasing when doing HCG.

10. Sugar. Read your labels to make sure that you don't have any hidden sugars. They're sneaky about that stuff and it has more than 99 different names! Thirty of the names are:

- barley malt
- beet sugar
- brown sugar
- buttered syrup
- cane-juice crystals
- cane sugar
- caramel
- carob syrup
- corn syrup
- corn syrup solids
- date sugar
- dextran
- dextrose
- diatase
- diastatic malt
- ethyl maltol
- fructose
- fruit juice
- fruit juice concentrate
- glucose
- glucose solids
- golden sugar
- golden syrup
- grape sugar
- high-fructose corn syrup
- honey
- invert sugar
- lactose
- malt syrup
- maltodextrin
- maltose
- mannitol
- molasses
- raw sugar
- refiner's syrup
- sorbitol
- sorghum syrup
- sucrose
- sugar
- turbinado sugar
- yellow sugar

If you're spot on following the protocol, those are some of the trouble places that I've learned (some, the hard way) to ferret out.

Cocoa

Chocolate Strawberry Crème
20 drops NOW Foods Dark Chocolate Stevia
1t Walden Farms Strawberry jelly
1t Walden Farms Marshmallow Dip
20 oz hot water
Mix all ingredients together in 20oz mug. Add an additional dollop of marshmallow, if you'd like!

Raspberry Cocoa
1t Walden Farms Raspberry jelly
25 drops NOW Foods Dark Chocolate Stevia
20 oz hot water
1 dollop Walden Farms Marshmallow Dip
Mix jelly, stevia, and water together. Put dollop of marshmallow on top and enjoy!

White Dark Cocoa
30 drops NOW Foods Dark Chocolate Stevia
20 oz hot water
Mix all ingredients together in 20oz mug. Add an additional dollop of Walden Farms marshmallow, if you'd like!

Orange Cocoa
20 drops NOW Foods Dark Chocolate Stevia
8 drops orange Stevia
1T Orange peel
20 oz hot water
Mix stevia, orange peel, and water together.

Peppermint Cocoa
20 drops NOW Foods Dark Chocolate Stevia
10 drops Peppermint Stevia
20 oz hot water
Mix stevia, and water together. You might want to add a dollop of Walden Farms Marshmallow Dip to the top so it looks festive!

Coffee

Mocha Frappè

12oz of fresh brewed coffee

5 drops NOW Foods Dark Chocolate Stevia

1t Walden Farms Marshmallow Dip

6 ice cubes

Put all ingredients into blender and blend until smooth. Pour into 20 oz glass and enjoy.

French Vanilla Coffee

16oz of fresh brewed coffee

5 drops NOW Foods French Vanilla Stevia

1t Walden Farms Marshmallow Dip

In 16 oz coffee cup, add stevia and marshmallow dip first. Pour hot coffee over the top of that so it mixes while you're pouring. This is a great drink to have on your way out the door to work.

Raspberry Mocha

16 oz fresh brewed coffee

5 drops chocolate raspberry stevia

1T milk

In 16 oz coffee cup, add stevia and milk. Pour hot coffee over that so it mixes while you're pouring.

Caramel Mocha

16 oz fresh brewed coffee

1t Walden Farms Caramel dipping sauce

1T milk

In 16 oz coffee cup, add caramel and milk. Pour hot coffee over that so it mixes while you're pouring.

Caramel Mocha Frappè

20 oz fresh brewed coffee

1t Walden Farms Caramel dipping sauce

1t Walden Farms Marshmallow Dip

1T milk

6-10 ice cubes

Put all ingredients into blender and blend until smooth. Pour into 20 oz glass and enjoy.

Vanilla Toffee Coffee

16 oz fresh brewed coffee

5 drops vanilla stevia

5 drops toffee stevia

1T milk

In 16 oz coffee cup, add stevia and milk. Pour hot coffee over that so it mixes while you're pouring.

Tea

Fairy Rooibus

2T loose leaf Rainbow Rooibus tea

1/4t organic lavender

8 drops stevia

Put all ingredients into your tea pot, fill with water that's just reached the boiling point and let steep 3-5 minutes. I like to drink this one hot in the mornings. It takes the edge off a hungry tummy in the beginning of the Protocol.

Vanilla Rooibus Crème

2T loose leaf Rooibus tea

10 drops NOW Foods French Vanilla Stevia

1t Walden Farms Marshmallow Dip

1T milk

Put all ingredients into your tea pot, fill with water that's just reached the boiling point and let steep 3-5 minutes. Be sure to stir before pouring to make sure all ingredients are fully mixed.

Chocolate Mint Tea

2T loose leaf Mint tea

10 drops NOW Foods Dark Chocolate Stevia

1T milk

Put all ingredients into your tea pot, fill with water that's just reached the boiling point and let steep 3-5 minutes.

Vanilla Mint Tea

2T loose leaf Mint tea

10 drops NOW Foods French Vanilla Stevia

1T milk

Put all ingredients into your tea pot, fill with water that's just reached the boiling point and let steep 3-5 minutes.

Vanilla Orange Rooibus

2T loose leaf Rooibus tea

1T dried orange rind

10 drops NOW Foods French Vanilla Stevia

Put all ingredients into your tea pot, fill with water that's just reached the boiling point and let steep 3-5 minutes.

Note: Any of these can be iced for a cool refreshing drink on a hot day.

Savory Drinks

Vegetable Broth
38 calories

2c water
1T vegetable bullion
1t parsley flakes
10 fennel seeds
salt & pepper to taste
2c celery (38 calories)

Bring all ingredients except the celery to a boil. Puree celery and add to boiling broth. Allow to simmer 10 minutes so the flavors mix. Serve hot or over ice.

Savory Tomato Sipper
65 calories

1c tomatoes (65 calories)
1T tomato paste
2c water
1T vegetable bullion
1/2t garlic
salt & pepper to taste

Bring water, tomato paste, bullion, garlic, salt & pepper to boil. Puree tomatoes and add to boiling broth. Allow to simmer 10 minutes so the flavors mix. Serve hot or over ice.

Basil Broth

2c water
1T tomato paste
1t basil
1t italian seasoning
1 clove garlic, minced
1T vegetable bullion

Bring all ingredients to a boil, then turn down the heat and allow to simmer 10 minutes more. Serve hot.

Of Habits & Hangups...

We just hooked our satellite TV back up after it was off for the whole summer. With the TV came some of the old habits that I developed when it was on during last autumn/winter/spring. That includes the urge to munch while it's on. Luckily for me, I was *aware* of it when it happened and checked with my body to see if I was actually hungry or if this was just something that was externally triggered.

It was external. :)

And I knew it.

That's MOST of the battle, right?

So, I decided to go ahead and search for some articles about breaking bad habits... Here's what I found - I hope it helps us all:

"Good habits are hard to develop but easy to live with" and "Bad habits are easy to develop but hard to live with", according to Brian Tracey, a well-known motivational teacher. You may recognize that to successfully manage habit changes, breaking bad habits may be required in order to develop new ones.

Breaking bad habits takes at least 21 days. Of course, in difficult cases, it can take as long as a year. Here's an example of the process of how to change an unhealthy habit to a healthy habit. Suppose you've decided that coffee is not good for you and right now, you drink coffee with sugar daily. The new habit you would like to institute is to drink herbal tea without sugar.

At first, it may be challenging to break the bad habit of drinking coffee. You will have to use self-discipline for the first few weeks but gradually it will get easier. Once you are able to change the old habit to a new healthier one, it will serve you very well. Habits are remarkable because they don't require thinking. You just "do it" for years until you find yourself changing the habit again.

Here are 5 easy steps for changing habits:

1. Awareness: You must become aware of your habits. What is this habit exactly? How is this bad habit or group of bad habits affecting you? How is this habit affecting others? For example, smoking often has negative effects on others as well as on you.

2. Wanting to Change: As someone with a health problem, you must decide that breaking bad habits

through a conscious effort is a worthy goal. You must convince yourself that the change in the habit is worth the effort involved.

3. Commitment: You must be determined to do whatever it takes for breaking bad habits so that you can better control your life. You make a decision that "no matter what" you will change the habit. You do the work required to stop. Here are some examples of habits you might want to change: Smoking, eating too much, eating processed foods, not exercising, drinking coffee or other beverages with caffeine in them, eating too much sugar or fat, drinking alcohol, procrastinating, etc.

4. Consistent Action: It is important to focus on changing just one habit at a time. Then, take consistent daily actions for breaking the bad habit that has been causing problems and take the actions to develop a new one. We suggest doing this process one step at a time rather than trying to do it all at once. Sometimes changing a habit can be done "cold turkey" like smoking and sometimes it works better to make a gradual change.

Be sure to give yourself positive rewards often for taking small actions toward changing a bad habit. Continual day-by-day actions are what are critical. This is NOT about an occasional action or step. It is about being consistent every day.

5. Perseverance: There will be times when you question whether it is all worth it. You'll say to yourself that breaking these bad habits is too difficult; that you are too "weak" to change. Your old self, often so comfortable living with the bad habits, is trying to hold on. Breaking your old patterns may require meditation and prayer.

Visualize regularly the rewards for following through and the costs of not following through on breaking the bad habits and especially the value to your future of building new better habits.

Get support from others, especially other people who want to make changes in their lives and read about people who have been successful in breaking bad habits. Affirm that, no matter what, you will not backslide into your old bad habit patterns.

Now, you are armed with a 5-step process for breaking any bad habit or other condition that requires changing. If you have an addiction to something such as alcohol, these steps alone may not be enough. You may require additional professional help or a support group, but for most cases this 5-step process will do the trick!

T. McDonald is a lifelong student of inner growth and a writer. She edits Diabetes Guide where you will find information on the glycemic index diet, weight loss, diets, managing diabetes, alternative sweeteners, breast cancer bracelets, how to prevent breast cancer and much more.

Printed with Permission, Copyright 2005 T. McDonald

In making another dish, the Buffalo Chips with the side of Waldorf Salad, we decided that we needed to make a soup using some of the elements of that dish. There's a full set of flavor layering in this soup that we're sure you're going to fall in love with on the first chill day you have to sit in a window seat, sip this wonderful clear soup and envision yourself at the end of your HCG Journey.

Buffalo Celery Soup
139 calories

2 green onion, sliced really thin, about 2" of the white part
1T fresh horse radish, minced
100g buffalo (100 calories)
2 cloves garlic, minced
salt
Mix all ingredients together and set aside to allow flavors to mix.

3c water
1 large bay leaf
2T beef bullion
2c celery (39 calories)
2 tips of green onions (the white part only), sliced really thin
Bring water, bay leaf, bullion, green onion to boil. Make 18 meatballs, 1t each, and drop them into the boiling water to cook for 10 minutes. Add celery and allow to cook for an additional 10 minutes. Serve hot with a grissini stick.

Lest you all think I'd leave you hanging for lunch menus (And I may someday! ACK! You'll all be lunch repeaters!), Jackie sent pictures for her buffalo chili so I can post them today. Hurray! It sounds like a wonderfully easy recipe that could be done at work, provided you cooked the buffalo first. It would make everyone sooo jealous. :) They'll all want to be on HCG with you.

Buffalo Chili

175 calories

Chef: Jackie R, Winner of Main Dish Recipe Contest

100 gr Ground Buffalo (100 calories)

1 c tomato cut into bite sized pieces (65 calories)

1 1/2 t minced garlic

1/2 t cumin

1/2 t oregano

1 chicken bouillion cube

1/2 t chili powder (more if you like spicier)

dash of red pepper flakes or ground red pepper

1/2 t onion powder

salt and pepper to taste

1 cup water

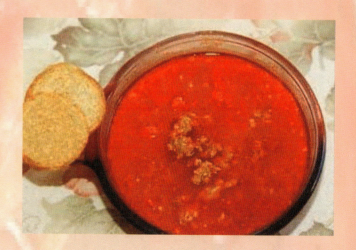

Dry fry ground buffalo till almost cooked, add to crock pot. Add all rest ingredients to crock pot and let cook until done.

Buffalo Chips
100 calories

2 green onion, sliced really thin, about 2" of the white part
1T fresh horse radish, minced
100g buffalo (100 calories)
2 cloves garlic, minced
salt
Mix all ingredients together and set aside to allow flavors to mix.

Sauce:
1/4c ketchup (see the Staple Sauces list)
2T Worcester (see the Staple Sauces list)
1 1/2t Plochman's Stone Ground Mustard (or Dijon)
8 drops Toffee Stevia
1 1/2t water
1 1/2t garlic butter (made with Butter Buds)
salt & pepper to taste
Mix all these ingredients and set aside to allow flavors to mingle.

Broth:
2c water
1 large bay leaf
1T beef bullion
Bring broth to a boil. Make 18 meatballs, 1t each, and drop them into the boiling water to cook for 10 minutes and remove. Place meatballs into a ramekin and pop them into the oven, uncovered, at 375* for 15 minutes. Cover ramekin with foil and return to oven for an additional 15 minutes.

Chef's Note: There's enough sauce in this recipe for twice as many meatballs as this recipe makes. You'll need to either freeze the remaining sauce or double the meatball section of the recipe and freeze the whole meal for eating lunch out at work.

Buffalo Meatballs and Sour Kraut

100 calories

Meatballs:
1 t onion flakes
salt and pepper to taste
100 ground buffalo (100 calories)

Sauce:
1/4 c ketchup (see Staple Sauces list)
1/2 T tomato paste
2 drop toffee stevia
3 drops Tabasco
1 T milk
1/4 t. butter buds (makes everything better)
chili powder to taste
salt and pepper

sour kraut

Make a stock of 2c water and 1T beef bouillon, bring to a boil. Mix meatball ingredients and form balls. Add buffalo meatballs to boiling stock and cook about 10 minutes.
Mix the other ingredients (except sour kraut) together and set aside.
Put meatballs into bottom of oven proof dish, cover them with sauce, then cover all that with kraut. Bake for 30 - 40 minutes at 375 degrees.

Buffaloaf
127 calories

Meatloaf:

100g ground buffalo (100 calories)

1/3 cup grated zucchini (7 calories)

1 grissini breadstick, pulverized (20 calories)

1T milk

1/4t italian seasoning

1/4t garlic powder

1/4t onion powder

a sprinkle of celery seeds

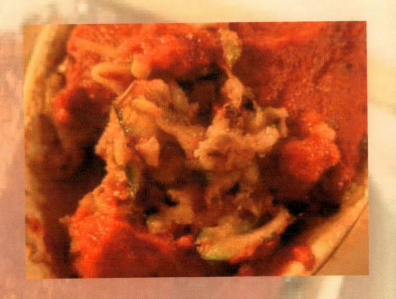

Sauce:

1T tomato paste

1/8t onion powder

1/8t garlic powder

1/8t italian seasoning

1/8t fennel seed

1 drop stevia

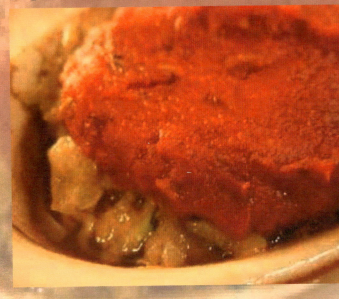

Mix meat ingredients together and pat into a patty. Place in center of 8" foil and set aside. Combine sauce ingredients together in bowl and spread on top of patty. Make foil into pocket and cook buffaloaf 45 minutes at 350* (toaster ovens work good for this if you don't want to heat the whole house). Uncover buffaloaf and broil patty 10 minutes. Then serve it HOT HOT HOT!

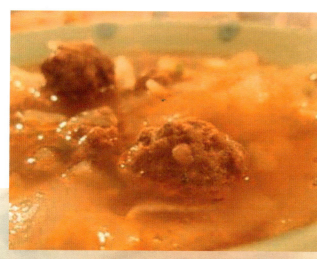

I've found a new favorite meat. It took me a looooonnnngggg time to try it, but it tastes like a really great cut of beef to me. I buy it organic, just so you know. It's one of the only meats that I do buy organic, because I've heard that the flavor of buffalo can really be terrible or can be a real treat, depending on what's added to the meat during processing. An organic meat is the purest I can find, other than taking a buffalo down myself for supper. We've got buffalo and onions and a little heat to the dish. I think you're going to LOVE it.

Running with the Buffalo

161 calories

100g buffalo (100 calories)
1c mayan sweet onion (61 calories)

3c water
1t jalapeno
1/4t chili powder
1T beef bullion
2 1/2T southwest seasoning (divided)
1 1/2t cumin
3 cloves fresh garlic, minced (divided)
1t onion powder
salt & pepper to taste

In pan, add water, jalapeno, chili powder, bullion, 1 1/2T southwest seasoning, cumin, 1/2 the minced garlic, salt and pepper to taste. Bring to a boil. While the broth is heating, add buffalo, 1T southwest seasoning, remaining garlic, onion powder, and a shake or two of salt & pepper to a bowl. Mix this well together and form 1" meatballs.

When broth is boiling, carefully add meatballs one at a time so as not to splash. Turn heat down to a simmer and let sit 10 minutes. Add onion and let simmer an additional 20 minutes, then serve hot.

The longer you simmer, the more the flavors mingle. Just don't let it simmer so long that the onions get mushy.

This particular recipe is one that is ***very*** close to my all time favorite meal in the whole world. My Mom's Barley Soup. I would rather have that soup than anything available to me, including fettuccine or fondue! And I really love cheese, too.

I never knew how to make the broth and always just begged Mom to make it. It's sort of like her brownies. Where I've never made a pan of it, it's one of those memories from childhood that just shouldn't be messed with as an adult. It's the perfect feel-good food. A whole body full of great feelings gets served up with each spoonful that touches your lips.

There's no pictures of this soup just yet – last time I made it, I could only think about getting that soup into my mouth and getting those great feelings zipping around! I think my family actually liked me better after I ate it.

I couldn't stop smiling.

Tomato Basil Soup
165 calories

100g buffalo (100 calories)
2c water
1T beef bullion
1t basil
1t onion flakes
2 cloves garlic, minced
1T tomato paste
salt & pepper to taste
1c tomatoes (65 calories)

Bring water, bullion, basil, onion, garlic, tomato paste to a boil. Add ground buffalo and allow to cook. Turn heat down, add tomato and allow soup to simmer 10 minutes. Serve hot and enjoy!

It's Never Been This Easy...

It's Never Been This Easy
(Because it truly hasn't)
By Guest Blogger, "Chris"

Here's the thing.

This protocol is not hard to understand. There are a few basic rules.

1. Know when to take your HCG drops and how much and be consistent. It is the key to the program. Three times a day, morning, noon and night....10 - 45 minutes before consuming a meal.
2. Eat only what's on the list of approved foods.
3. Eat only the approved amounts. Weigh out the meats, measure the vegetables.
4. Do not mix your meats or vegetables. So you have chicken and zucchini for dinner. Not chicken and zucchini and tomatoes!
5. DRINK WATER!!
6. Weigh every day and measure once a week on the same day each week. Watch the weight drop and the inches vanish.

You can get as creative as you like within the regimen of foods allowed. Add spices and other "no sugar, no fat" products that have been approved on the diet and keep yourself satisfied. It takes a little effort but it's worth it.

Folks, this is your body. Why mess with it if you aren't serious about it? This diet program will work but you need to know what you are doing before starting it so you can be prepared to succeed. If you do it right, you will not have cravings or be hungry.

If you just can't wrap your mind around the program, then don't bother! You will be wasting your time and money.

For some of you, this is just another opportunity to fail and you are doing a good job of it. You can make up any excuse for not succeeding. Don't let this be just another diet that wasn't convenient or didn't fit into your lifestyle. It's way too easy to sabotage yourself that way and never lose the weight that is weighing you down.

This is the easiest program I have ever been on and it works and promises to help you remain at a weight you can really live with. Please! Don't treat this Protocol the same way you have treated every other failed diet in your life. It doesn't have to be that way! Get your head in the game! 'This program is designed on a 28, 40 or 60 day "round." You can live on 500 calories a day for (at the minimum) 28 days. You CAN follow those few simple, albeit strict rules for 28 days. YOU CAN DO IT! At the end of that period you will be slimmer and no doubt... healthier.

So, get serious.

Know what you are doing to your body and prepare yourself emotionally to DO this. Consider this your kick in the butt and MOVE!

If you need help and support then of course reach out. If you are one of those that has until now just decided to diet the HCG way and haven't done your homework then do it now. All the information you need is on Jayme's blog and she is happy to help you but get the knowledge you need.

Don't wait! It's your body, your story, and your responsibility to yourself.

An old favorite in my family during the autumn change is cream of broccoli soup. Basically, the ingredients we normally use follow the protocol, so it was just a matter of reducing the regular amounts used for a whole family down to the recipe for one. I didn't quite get there and the recipe that follows is enough for two. So, make one for yourself today and freeze the other to take with you to work tomorrow and warm up all morning in your wee little crock pot. Everyone will be soooo jealous - I promise!

Autumn Bliss Soup
160 calories per serving

100g chicken (110 calories per serving)
2c broccoli (50 calories per serving)
2c water
2T chicken bouillon
2T onion, chopped (large if you're really really strict about not mixing veggies)
2T milk
1t celery seed
1 or 2 bay leaves
1T butter buds

Chop up broccoli so that each floret is divided into about 5 pieces and keep the stalk. Steam the broccoli so it's about half done. Take off the stove and add 3/4 of this to the blender and puree it completely. Cut the remaining 1/4 of the broccoli into spoon size bites and set aside. To your soup pan, bring water, bouillon, onion, milk, celery seed, bay leaves and butter buds to a boil. Pound chicken thin and slice into bite sized pieces, add to soup pan. When chicken is cooked completely, add all the broccoli to the soup pan and let simmer 15 minutes.

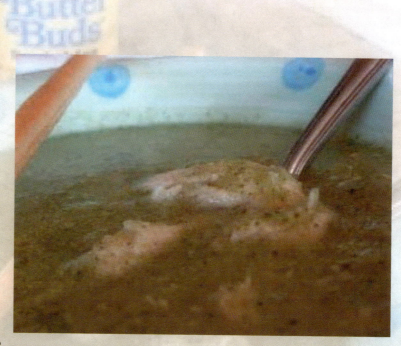

Immediately pull out the bay leaves or they'll just continue to get strong in the soup. At this point, you could also pull out the onion, too. Serve hot.

Asian Garlic Chicken

Last night's dinner was mostly compliments of Walden Farms, as far as taste goes. I found their salad dressings & ketchup in a store in Hood River, OR after visiting my nutritionalist, Tami, at Daniel's Health Store. (daniels@gorge.net). I bought my HCG there, picked up a few vitamins, and some different flavors of stevia.

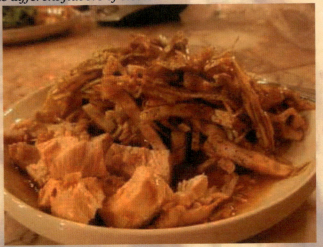

Anyway, I headed up to Rosauer's and found Walden Farms salad dressings on sale 2 for $6.

They were sold out of the one I really wanted, Dijon Honey, but I got one of each of all the rest. Asian, Ranch, Creamy Bacon, 1000 Island, Balsamic, Raspberry Vinegrette, and Bleu Cheese. I went searching then for the Ketchup. It wasn't on sale, but it was there! :)

When I got home, I immediately pulled out the chicken I was planning to have but had no idea what to do with. I also grabbed some cabbage and talked my Mom into trying the salad dressings with me last night. She often helps me come up with recipes and taste tests them with me. But I'm getting ahead of myself.

Asian Garlic Chicken
110 calories

100g chicken

2T Walden Farms Asian dressing

1 clove fresh garlic, minced

In center of 8" foil, place chicken, top with garlic and spread Asian dressing over all of it. Fold into packet and allow to marinate in frig at least 1 hour. Put in 350* oven for 25 minutes or until chicken is done.

We served this up on two separate plates. One (mine) had cabbage tossed with the Walden Farms Balsamic dressing. The other (Mom's) had spinach tossed with the Walden Farms Creamy Bacon dressing.

Mom reported that the dressings mingled very nicely together and that if she were working outside the home, she'd probably make the chicken up the night before, take the spinach and Creamy Bacon salad dressing (in separate containers), warm up the chicken at lunch time and just dump it all over the top of the spinach. Just a thought.

Today's lunch turned out to be a delightful concoction I created on the fly. I told you all that I'm just getting bored with the same old same old sorts of recipes, right? Well, I put some things together today that I never would've considered before. It's kind of funny, too, because one of the ingredients contains another of the ingredients that I used, so it was a natural marriage. I just never considered it before.

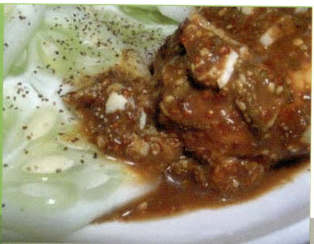

Balsamic Mustard Chicken

110 calories

100g chicken (110 calories)

2T Balsamic Vinegar

2T Stone Ground mustard (I use Plochman's)

3 cloves fresh garlic, chopped coarsely

2t dried basil

Mix all ingredients except chicken in a small bowl. Add chicken and cover on both sides with the marinade. Cover and let stand 1 hour in frig. Place chicken in ramekin and pour remaining marinade over the top of it. Bake in oven 20 minutes at 350*. When 20 minutes is done, pour 2T hot water over the chicken to dilute the marinade a little, then cook another 10 minutes. Take out of oven and cut chicken into bite sized pieces, then toss with marinade before transferring to your plate.

I served this with lemon cucumber (see the picture for what they look like) fresh from a neighbor's garden. I topped the cucumber with fresh ground pepper and dipped the slices into Walden Farms Ranch dressing but decided that I liked a little bite of the marinade and chicken on top of each cucumber best.

Barley soup is a family favorite the year round, but especially when it's cold outside. The leaves are changing on the trees right now and the winds are picking up, bringing promises of an early snow this year. This particular soup has the colors of early fall in it, which is why I like it so much during the autumn. It's like eating autumn. :)

This recipe makes it easy to enjoy a meal with your family, too. Cooking a separate meal for yourself and then one for your family is just silly. This recipe will let you make just one meal for everyone and they'll come back for seconds (I'm full after eating it and still wish I could go back for seconds or thirds)!

Bar the Barley Soup
110 calories

100g ground chicken (110 calories)
1/2t fresh minced garlic
1/4t basil
1/4t onion flakes
salt & pepper to taste
Mix in small bowl and set aside.

2 1/2c water
2t chicken boulion
1T tomato paste
1/2t minced fresh garlic
1/4t basil
1/4t minced onion
In pan, bring all ingredients to boil, drop meat mixture in by little small meatballs about as big as your thumbnail. Bring back to boil and then turn down and let simmer for 10 minutes. Chop up veggie, add to stock and cook until the veggie is done. The longer you cook the stock, the better flavor you'll get.

Chicken Celery Aspic
150 calories

100g chicken
4c water (divided)
1t rosemary
2 cloves minced garlic
a splash of Worcester sauce
1/4t chili powder
1t chicken tomato bullion
a splash of Tabasco sauce
salt and pepper to taste
2pkg Knox gelatin
2pkg stevia
1 bunch celery hearts
juice of a large lime

Pound chicken, put in 2c water, bring to boil. Add 1t rosemary, 2 cloves minced garlic, a splash of Worcester sauce, 1/4t chili powder, 1t chicken tomato bullion, a splash of Tabasco, salt and pepper to taste. Bring back to boil. Turn down to simmer, let simmer 20 minutes.

Remove chicken, cut into small pieces (smaller than bite sized), set aside. If you don't like spices in, you can strain them out at this point, but keep the broth. With hot broth, add 1 envelop Knox gelatin and stir until well dissolved. Add 4-5 ice cubes and stir. If it gels too fast, add a little cold water. Pour chicken into this mixture and pour into a mold or a 4x8 dish. Put that in the frig.

Chop 1 bunch celery hearts, very, very fine (less than 1/8 inch thick). Bring another 2c water to a boil, pour in another envelope of Knox gelatin and 2 pkg stevia. Stir until dissolved. Add another 4-5 ice cubes and juice of a whole large lime. Stir. If it gels too fast, add a little cold water to it. Add celery to this mixture.

Take the first chicken gelatin back out of the frig, it should be fairly solidified. Pour the celery mixture over the chicken and put it back in the frig and refrigerate until firmly gelled.

Chef's Notes: You could use cabbage, but it should be shredded before you add it to the gelatin mixture.

Chicken Sausage
110 calories

100g ground chicken breast (110 calories)
1T garlic
1/2t red chili pepper flakes
2t sage
1/8t fennel seed
1t thyme
1/4t cinnamon
Mix all ingredients together and dry fry as patties. OR, for a really great treat, try the recipe below.

Savory Stuffed Apple
200 calories

100g ground chicken (110 calories)
1T chicken bullion
1 apple (90 calories)
1/4t cinnamon
1/8t lemon juice
4 drops stevia
dash pumpkin pie spice
salt to taste
Wash apples and cut the top off them, 1" from the top. Scoop out the inside of the apple, leaving about 1/2 inch of the apple along the sides. Chop up the flesh from the apple middle and add to a small bowl. Add chicken, bullion, cinnamon, lemon juice, stevia, pumpkin pie spice, and salt to the apples and mix thoroughly. Stuff apple shells with chicken mixture, place apple top on the mixture and bake 30minutes at 350*. Serve hot with a side salad of romaine hearts!

Chicken Tomato Soup-erior
175 calories

100g chicken (110 calories)

1c tomatoes (65 calories)

2c water

1/2t cumin

1/4t oregano

1/4t red pepper flakes

1/8t ground cloves

1/4t jalapeno (diced fine)

2t chicken bullion

salt to taste

Boil all ingredients (except the tomatoes) until chicken is cooked through. Cut up tomatoes (fresh off the vine is best!) and add to soup sized bowl. Remove chicken and cut into small pieces, add to tomatoes. Ladle broth onto chicken and tomatoes. Let cool off a little and use your grissini breadstick to cool your tongue as you enjoy this dish.

Tonight's supper is a quick one and could be made in a small crock pot at work, if you needed to! It's easy peasy and very filling.

Chili Tomato Chicken
175 calories

- 100g chicken (110 calories)
- 3c water
- 1T southwest seasoning
- 2T chicken tomato boullion
- 2t cumin
- 1t onion powder
- 1t garlic powder
- 1/2t chili powder
- Allowed amount of tomato (1 cup=65 calories)

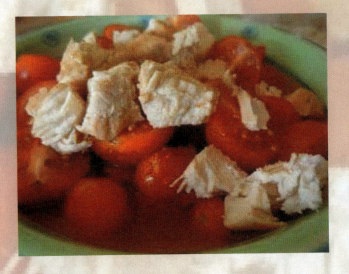

In pan, add chicken, water, spices and bring to a boil. Allow chicken to cook. While chicken is cooking, cut tomatoes into bite size pieces and add to a soup bowl. When chicken is fully cooked, pour broth and chicken over tomatoes. Serve immediately!

Today's lunch was a great success. I'm sure you're all going to love it, but it does take a little planning so the chicken marinates overnight in the sauce. I think it would be great with steak or roast beef, too!

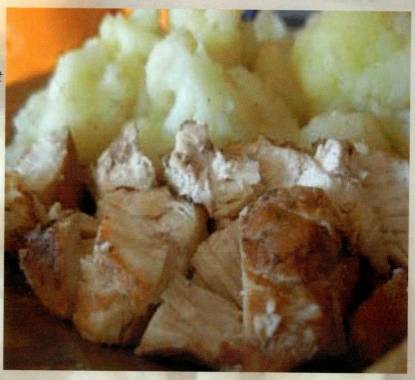

Cola Chicken

110 calories

100g chicken (110 calories)

1 can of Cola Zevia

4 large garlic cloves

1T Worcester (see the Staple Sauces list)

1t liquid smoke

1/4t chili powder

1/4t salt

3 drops Valencia Orange Stevia

1/2 onion cut, into half rings

Put everything except the chicken into a bowl and mix thoroughly. Place chicken in the marinade, cover, and refrigerate over night. Cook at 350* for 30 minutes or until done!

Yesterday went much better than I thought it was going to. After our cello lesson, we (my family and I) planned to head over to a McDonalds with a play place thing so the kids could play and run off some of that pent up energy from driving 2 hours, then sitting to play instruments for 2 hours.

First, though, we needed to get some supplies. I realized, after looking through my list of recipes that I have not had a *single* salad while following this protocol. That's saying something about recipe creativity, considering salads are supposed to be "diet food." Hahahaha!

Anyway, we headed out to Fred Meyer's and I ran in to get a bag of lettuce. Mom was having a salad, too, but she wanted a spinach salad after being so sick (she & the kids had the flu). So, I grabbed up a bag of romaine lettuce hearts, a box of baby spinach, and four oranges. I ran through the self check out and paid for them all, then ran back out to the rig.

When we got to McDonalds, Mom went in with the kids and ordered their lunch (we don't often eat there because it's sooooo not good for the body - normally, we go to Subway). While she was doing that, I grabbed up a Zevia, my salad dressing, a breadstick, and the Cola Chicken made the night before and headed into the restraunt. Found the ideal seat so we could watch the kids play and only then did I realize that I didn't have a bowl to eat out of. I looked around for something that I could use as a make-shift bowl and thought of the lid to the spinach. It was an inverse bowl, though, so that was not an option. :(

So, I opened the middle of the back of the bag, so it sort of acted like a bowl. I put the chicken on the romaine hearts and added my Walden Farms Asian dressing and *poof* I had a salad! The only thing missing, in my estimation, was cheese. ::grins:: I'm looking forward to Phase 3 just so I can have cheese.

Mom brought a cup of ice and I poured my Zevia into it, so it looked like I was drinking a "regular" soda, just like everyone else. Of course, mine was much more healthy and, therefore, I think it tastes better.

I didn't take pictures. I completely forgot my camera at home. Trying to remember to feed dogs, bring music, cello, recycling, get the kids their music and instruments, grab a notebook for doodling, all the food for following my protocol, and getting it all out to the car is quite a feat. The camera didn't even cross my mind until I was sitting there, ready to eat.

Anyway, it was much easier than I thought it would be, even without a proper bowl. And, as it was the first salad I've had in nearly 40 days, I think the creative minds of Less of Me is doing well!

I was a supper repeater last night when we got home. I made up the Buffaloaf recipe the night before and just needed to heat it up. Almost as soon as I was finished eating, I went to bed. I didn't even offer to help with the dishes or get a desert made up.

How rude of me, right?

*****

This morning, I got on the scale and saw one less number than I did yesterday, too! :)

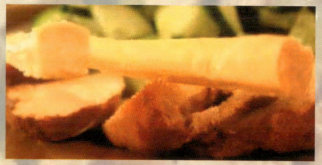

Tonight's supper is a test for Saturday. Saturday, we all head to Portland for cello, guitar, and piano lessons. I don't want to risk getting up there to the city and not being able to find what I need to have for lunch. And maybe for dinner, too.

So, I'm planning to do the recipe below for lunch and to make the meatloaf for supper. I think. Anyway, regardless of what I come up with, YOU get to have the recipe!

Cucumber Chicken Salad

139 calories

100g chicken (110 calories)

1 1/2c water

1T chicken boullion

4T loose leaf vanilla mint tea

5 cloves garlic, chopped

salt to taste

1T whole dried rosemary

2c cucumber (29 calories)

Put chicken into pot with everything except the cucumber and cook over medium heat until done. Refrigerate overnight.

When it's time for the meal to be eaten, chop up the cucumber, top with the chicken and use Walden Farms dressing (the Chef recommends either Honey Dijon or Asian).

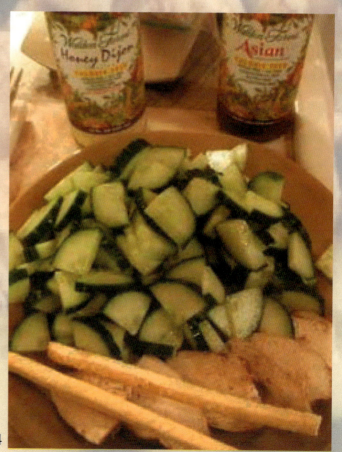

Herb Marinated Chicken

Today, I'm a lunch repeater. I really wanted Herb the Halibut, as it's one of my favorites and it's so easy to make. When you just aren't hungry, then you look at the clock and you realize it's time to eat NOW, this is a fast one to throw together. It helps that I had halibut already thawed in the frig, too. Not to leave you all in a lurch though for something new to try, I have this recipe that I've been intending to try out, but I don't have any tarragon vinegar made up yet. :(Maybe you do? If you do and decide to try this one out, please let me know how it turns out, and if I need to adjust any of the spices along the way.

I suppose this would work on just about any of the meats that we're allowed, but I think it goes especially well on the chicken...

Herb Marinated Chicken
110 calories

100g chicken (110 calories)

2T tarragon vinegar

dash of soy sauce

1/4t parsley

1 bay leaf

1/4t basil

1/4t oregano

pinch mustard

salt & pepper to taste

Combine all spices in a small bowl. Coat chicken well. Cover the mixture and refrigerate overnight. Heat oven to 350* and bake 45 minutes or until chicken is done.

Chicken and Tomatoes

So, tonight, I figured it was time to just sort of be lazy about dinner. Hehehe. I already had the chicken out thawing, so figured I'd better use it. What can you do with chicken that'll make it taste yummy and in a rush? Well, I used the recipe we normally use for fried chicken, but without the flour. Since the spices are allowed, this should result in at least the taste of fried chicken. And, really, that's all I'm after anyway, right?

Lazy Sunday Chicken
110 calories

100g chicken (110 calories)
1/8t paprika
1/8t garlic powder
1/8t salt
a shake of pepper
stick of cinnamon

In center of 8" foil, place chicken. One at a time, in order above, sprinkle chicken with spices on both sides. Add cinnamon stick on top of chicken, cover with foil and put in oven (or toaster oven) on 350* for 40 minutes or until done.
I've got some beautiful steak tomatoes waiting for me to do something with. I think, tonight, in honor of Lazy Sunday, I'm going to just slice 'em up, salt 'em, and eat 'em.

Tip

It turns out that when we crave chocolate, we aren't actually craving the chocolate, per se. Rather, we're craving the magnesium that's in it. Since chocolate is definitely off the Protocol, add a couple of magnesium tablets to your diet a few days before your cycle and all throughout your cycle. You shouldn't have the craving for that sweet confection any more.

For this dish, the only thing you're going to regret is the end of the bowl. Very flavorful, wonderfully filling, and definitely a taste of Japan. Originally, this dish, Won Ton Soup, is made with water chestnuts, ground pork, and won tons. Won tons are thin little 5" square noodles that you wrap around the meatball before you put it into the boiling broth to cook. Won means "swallowing a cloud." The cloud in our dish is more from the spinach, but don't let that dissuade you! It's still as delightful as the original!

Non Ton Soup

123 calories

Part One:
2 1/2c water
1T chicken bouillon
1T Soy sauce (more if desired)
Bring to boil.
Part Two:
100g ground chicken (110 calories)
White part of two green onions, cut *very thin*
1 1/2t minced fresh ginger
Mix meatballs and drop into boiling broth and allow to cook, about 20 minutes.
Part Three:
Allowed amount of spinach (2c=13calories)
Wash spinach, then hold spinach really tight together and cut into 1/2" strips. After meatballs are cooked, add spinach and let simmer 10 minutes. Serve hot with a grissini on the side and a cup of green tea for a traditional Japanese feel.
Chef's Note: This would be really terrific with mushrooms, too!

Orange Chicken Stir-Fry
110 calories

100g chicken, cut up (110 calories)
2T Bragg's Liquid Aminos
2c cabbage
1/4c water
8 drops orange stevia
1t Knox gelatin
1/8t salt
1/4t ground ginger

In medium skillet, sauté chicken in Bragg's over medium high heat for a few minutes until almost done. Add cabbage and fry for another two minutes. Mix all remaining ingredients together well in a glass and be sure to get the Knox gelatin well dissolved, without lumps. Reduce heat to medium, add sauce mix, and cover for about 5 minutes. Sauce should be thickened to a nice glaze when done.

Lunch today was a different sort of dish - variety is the spice of life, after all! I really like pounding the meat and putting it in the ramekin, as it makes the meat more able to soak up the flavors as well as making it more tender. I also used the grissini stick in this recipe and it gave a nice texture to it.

Orange Ginger Chicken
190 calories

1 orange (60 calories)
1/4t fresh ground ginger (up to 1/2t, depending on your taste)
1 or 2 drops stevia
1T stone ground mustard (Plochman's)
1T soy sauce
1/4t onion powder
salt & pepper to taste
1 grissini bread stick, crushed into a powder (20 calories)
100g chicken (110 calories)

Cut both the top and bottom of the orange off so there's about an inch left of the orange inside both ends. With the middle part of the orange, slice it into 4 pieces. It should cut the orange so it looks like the spokes of a wheel.

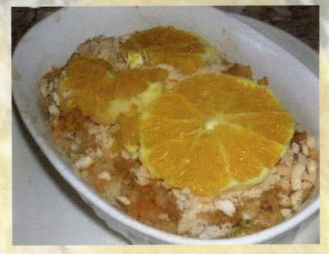

Take the two ends of the orange and squeeze the juice into a small bowl. Add ginger, stevia, mustard, and soy sauce to the juice of the orange. If there's not enough juice to make a runny sort of paste, then add a little water.

Pound chicken breast out so it's thin. In a separate bowl, add onion powder, salt, pepper, and grissini. Mix together. In ramekin, put two slices of the orange, lay chicken on top of that, cover with mustard mixture, pour bread stick mixture over that, then top with the last two slices of orange. Cover with foil and chill for 1 hour in frig. Cover with foil and bake at 350* for 20-25 minutes.

We found a local store with some of the Walden Farms products in it the night before we decided to make this and came up with this recipe. It's a great mix of tart and sweet and really gives a great finish.

Raspberry Mustard Chicken
130 calories

100g chicken (110 calories)
grissini stick (20 calories)
1T Walden Farms raspberry jelly
1T Plochman's Stone Ground Mustard
1/2t minced onions
1 clove garlic, minced
1/2t balsamic vinegar
1/4t chili powder
salt & pepper

Pound chicken until flat and set in ramekin. Crunch up grissini so there's both larger and smaller pieces, and set aside. In small bowl, mix jelly, mustard, onions, garlic, vinegar, chili powder, salt and pepper.

Pour jelly mixture over chicken, then sprinkle grissini stick on top. Place in oven at 350* for 30 minutes or until chicken is done.

This afternoon's lunch was absolutely fantastic!! I can't sing it's praises loud enough - **YOU MUST TRY THIS, EVEN IF YOU DON'T THINK YOU'D LIKE IT!!**

Savory Chicken & Apples
190 calories

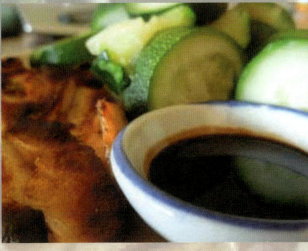

100g chicken (110 calories)

1 sliced apple (80 calories)

10 drops toffee stevia

1/8t salt

1/4t butter buds

just a sprinkle allspice

1t jalapeno

1T milk

Pound out chicken so it's very thin. Place chicken in bottom of a ramekin.

In small bowl, add stevia, salt, butter buds, allspice, jalapeno, milk and combine. Add apples to the mixture, then toss to fully coat them. Pour apple mixture on top of chicken in ramekin and bake 20 minutes at 350* then broil another 15 minutes. While cooking, make both the Garlic Zucchini and Balsamic Vinegar Sauce.

Garlic Zucchini (20 calories)

zucchini (1c=20 calories)

3 cloves garlic, cut in half

1t tomato-chicken bullion

Add bullion to water in steamer and bring to boil, add zucchini and garlic and allow to steam.

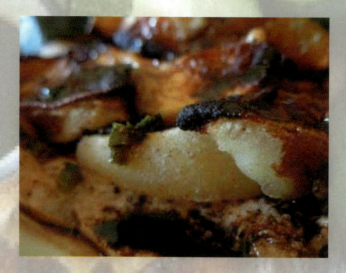

Balsamic Vinegar Sauce

1/4c balsamic vinegar

2 drops toffee stevia

Reduce this by putting it on the stove and bring it to a boil, then pick up the pan and swirl it around to check the viscosity. You want it thicker but not to cook it so long that it turns into a hard "candy."

When everything is ready, place apple chicken on one side of your plate, the zucchini on the other. Top the apple chicken with the Balsamic Vinegar Sauce and enjoy hot.

Chef's Note: If you are going to choose a different veggie, make sure you choose one that's pretty bland, as this dish has a LOT of flavor.

Sott'er celo de Roma

"On an evening in Roma..."

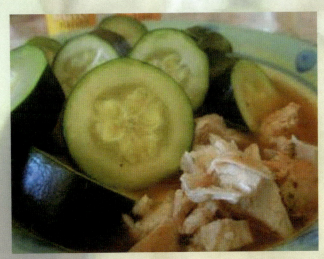

Today, we proclaimed it Italian day! Well, at least Italian lunch. :)

Zucchini and Italian Chicken - we forgot to play Dean Martin's Best while we were making it and eating, but upon reflection, we should have! It'd get us "in the mood."

So, I recommend a parmesean flavored Grissini to go along with your evening in Roma.

Sott'er celo de Roma

130 calories

100g chicken (110 calories)

Allowed amount Zucchini (1c=20 calories)

3c water

5 fresh basil leaves

2T tomato chicken bullion

1T Italian Seasonings

1t onion powder

1t garlic powder

In pot, add water and seasonings. Add chicken and allow to simmer until chicken is tender (about 30 minutes). Cut up zucchini into 1" rounds. In steamer, add zucchini and allow to steam for 20 minutes or until a fork will easily go through the flesh. Cut chicken into bite sized pieces and leave the broth in the pot to continue simmering. Place zucchini on plate (or bowl) and top with chicken. If you desire the broth (sauce), pour over everything. We topped it with both cheese and butter flavoring.

Delicious!

Como e bella ce la luna brille e strette
Strette como e tutta bella a passeggiare
Sotto il cielo di Roma

Down each avenue or via, street or strata
You can see 'em disappearing two by two
On an evening in Roma

Do they take 'em for Espresso
Yea, I guess so
On each lover's arm a girl I wish I knew
On an evening in Roma

Though there's grinning and mandolining
In sunny Italy
The beginning has just begun
When the sun goes down

So, please meet me in the plaza near your casa
I am only one and that is one too few
On an evening in Roma

Don't know what the country's coming to
But when in Rome do as the Romans do
Will you?
On an evening in Roma

Though there's grinning and mandolining
In sunny Italy
The beginning has just begun
When the sun goes down

Como e bella ce la luna brille e strette
Strette como e tutta bella a passeggiare
Sotto il cielo di Roma

Don't know what the country's coming to
But in Rome do as the Romans do
Will you?
On an evening in Roma
Sott'er celo de Roma
On an evening in Roma

Lyrics © CANZONI MODERNE CA MO

Up Town Chicken Soup

110 calories

100g chicken (110 calories)

1/4t onion powder

1/4t chicken bouillon

1 1/2c water

5 cloves garlic

fresh basil

Bragg's' Liquid Aminos

Allowed amount of broccoli

Add water, bouillon, chicken, onion, garlic, basil. Allow chicken to cook fully. Add broccoli and allow to cook. "Salt" with Bragg's' - but be careful not to add too much or it'll be too salty.

A Funny

Last night, I dreamed of mixing my veggies. I had salsa, ratatouille, vegetable soup with all the veggies in it, cucumber & tomato salad, salad with all the veggies...

When I awoke from the dream at 5:30 this morning, all I could do was laugh at myself. There weren't any veggies that aren't allowed on the protocol, like avocado, only the ones that we can have right now in Phase two. But I was mixing them! Bad, bad, bad! Shame on me!

~Jayme

Today, we've got a new recipe for you. Mom is brilliant with food and can make just about anything taste gourmet - she certainly did with this one!

Broccoli Fish Soup
150 calories

100g Halibut (100 calories)
broccoli (allowed amount) (50 calories per cup)
1 T chicken tomato bullion (find this in the Mexican section of your store)
3 c water
1/2 t garlic powder
1/2 t onion granules
1/2 t dried basil
2 T Bragg's' Liquid Aminos
1/4 t paprika
salt & pepper to taste (we didn't use any salt, though)

Bring garlic, onion, basil, & water almost to a boil. Add broccoli & cook about 5 minutes with lid on. Set halibut on top of broccoli, pour Bragg's over fish and sprinkle with paprika. Replace lid & cook about another 5 minutes. Add salt, pepper to taste and enjoy! We added a sea salt grissini as a side and found it complimented this dish very well.

Orange Roughy

I bet you thought this was going to be about an orange flavored something or other, didn't you? :)

It's not.

For lunch today, we are *very* pleased to bring you the best fish out on the market, Orange Roughy. We kept it simple, because if you do too much with fish, it just overpowers the delicate flavors and ruins it.

Buttery Orange Roughy
76 calories

100g Orange Roughy (76 calories)
1T lemon juice
2t butter buds
1/2t dill
1/2t salt

In ramekin, place orange roughy in middle. Pour lemon over the top of the fish, then sprinkle butter buds on, followed by dill and salt. Cover ramekin with foil and bake at 350* for 15 minutes.

We chose to eat this with a higher calorie vegetable, because it's so low in caloric value. To get to the half way mark of 250 calories for lunch, we had 1 1/2 cup fresh sliced tomato on the side. Salt and pepper those tomatoes and it's the perfect afternoon dish. It's light and doesn't make you feel loaded down for the rest of the afternoon.

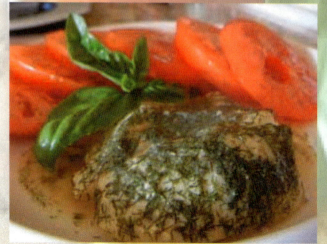

Lunch today is a simple dish, really. We're heading out to the pumpkin patch, so I'm short on time *again* when coming up for a lunch. It always happens that way when the kids are out of school and running circles around the adults! Ah, to have that sort of energy again. I have no idea what I'd do with it, but I'm sure I'd have less lists and more accomplished. So, it's a simple fish bake - always tasty and this fish doesn't taste fishy, so I'm really going to enjoy it.

Cod Bake
82 calories

100g cod (82 calories)
1t lemon juice
1/2t Celtic Sea Salt
1/2t dill weed
1/2t garlic powder (or, if you're like me and LIKE garlic, double this)
Place cod in ramekin, pour lemon juice over that. Sprinkle salt, dill, and garlic over it. Cover with foil and bake at 350* for 15 minutes or until flaky.

Movie Seats

This afternoon, my family went out to see Cloudy with a Chance of Meatballs. What a fun show! The last time I went to see a movie, my behind didn't want to fit in the seat. It's been that way for YEARS.

Today, I went in and was expecting the same *squished* feeling but my behind didn't even touch the sides of the chair!

WHOO HOOO!

There really is Less of Me!

Herb the Halibut

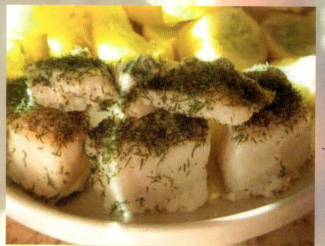

Tonight is a simple night to honor Herb. Herb, the Halibut, that is. We kept it simple so the seasonings wouldn't overwhelm the fragile flavors, broiling it just so the fish became flaky. We had it with a garlic grissini and summer squash.

Herb the Halibut
100 calories

100g halibut fillet (100 calories)

1/4 lemon

1t sea salt

1 clove fresh garlic, minced

1T dill weed

Rinse the fish and pat dry. Place in center of 8" square of foil and squeeze the juice from the lemon over the halibut. Season generously with salt first, then garlic, then the dill.

Broil about 8 minutes in toaster oven, until the fish is opaque and can be flaked with a fork. Keep in mind that your actual broiling time will vary with the thickness of your fish, so check often! Garnish with lemon slices. Serve with tomato slices, broccoli, or asparagus.

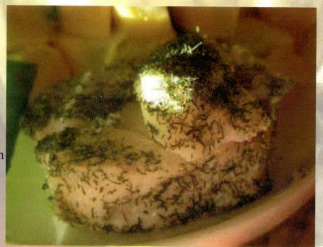

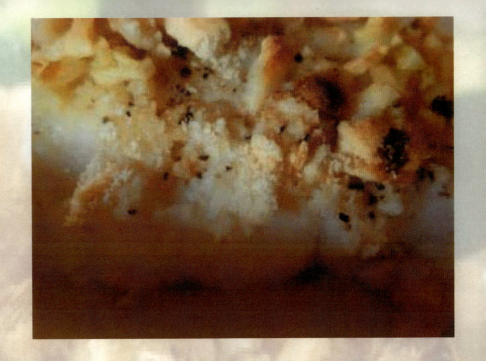

It's a Keeper!
(81 calories)

100g Orange Roughy (76 calories)
Garlic Butter (5 calories)
1 grissini stick
1t lime juice
salt & pepper to taste

In ramekin, place orange roughy in center. Squirt lime juice over the fish, then top with crunched up grissini stick (not pulverized into a powder - leave some chunks in there, too). Pour garlic butter over the grissini stick, then salt and pepper to taste. Bake at 350* for about 7 minutes or until fish flakes off with a fork.

Orange Roughy Soup

76 calories + your choice of veggie calories

100g orange roughy (76 calories)
2c water

1/2t fresh minced garlic
1/2t minced dry onion
1/8t thyme
1/8t basil
1/8t celery seed
1T tomato paste
1T chicken bouillon

Bring everything but the fish to a boil. Steam your veggie (mushrooms, celery, zucchini, spinach, green beans, yellow squash are best in this) separate. Add fish to the broth and let cook 10 minutes. Place veggie in your bowl and pour fish and broth over the top of it.

Apple Day

Drawn by Jayme Hunt of Sophisticated Sticks

Today is the sixth day of being on a plateau while on this protocol *and following it to the letter.* I figure that six days of being at the same weight makes it time for a shake down. Or maybe it's a shake up, I'm not sure. I think it's a shake down though, as I want to drop the weight rather than gain it. It's an apple day and I'll have apples coming out my ears!

My chosen apples are one of my all time favorites, Gala. I enjoy Honeykrisp and green (so they're tart) Golden Delicious. Mostly, I like all those because they have a nice satisfying crunch and an elegant sweetness followed directly with a tangy tart. It's a symphony in your mouth if you listen closely. I know what I'm talking about here because I grew up in AppleLand (Hood River Valley in Oregon) where the apples and pears grew everywhere there wasn't a house. I got so sick of them that I didn't eat them for a long time, in fact, because every time we were hungry as kids, Mom would tell us to eat an apple. :) It's kind of like oatmeal for me. We had oatmeal for breakfast nearly every day.

My memory of that could certainly be faulty, but about food, I recall vividly trying to choke down oatmeal that I was just so tired of eating it was making me green around the gills ("But it's good for you!") and apples coming out my ears.

The "Apple Day" concept feels a lot like that, but I'd rather feel like that than keep the weight on. :) Wish me luck!

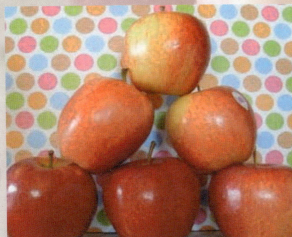
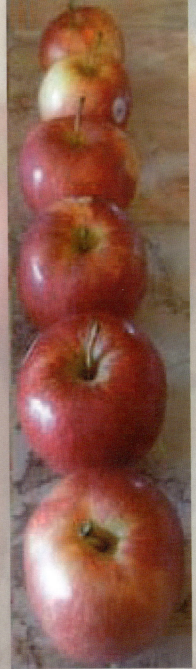

The beautiful, sunny French island of St. Barth is known the world over as the gastronomic capital of the Caribbean. Not that I've ever been there, but I've seen it in pictures and day dreamed about it - doesn't that count? Here is my HCG version of one of the tastiest and prettiest salads on the island. Bon Appetite!

St. Barth Seafood Salad
225 calories

Dressing
1/4 orange (save the rest for the salad part)
1T white vinegar
1T water
1/4t cloves
salt & pepper to taste

Salad
100g lobster (95 calories)
1 cup cabbage, sliced into strips (50 calories)
remainder of orange, cut into small cubes (60 calories)
1 sea salt grissini
To make dressing, put all dressing ingredients into blender on low speed until completely mixed. Refrigerate until ready to use.

In small bowl, place lobster and add 2T of the dressing and toss until lobster is coated. Place cabbage on plate then add the cubes of orange. Place lobster in the center atop the cabbage and orange, then serve with the remaining citrus vinaigrette on the side. Serve with grissini bread stick (20 calories), included in the whole dish caloric value) and fresh ground pepper.

I think I need a spell...

Maybe I need a spell to chase away the mean scale fairy I have in my house these days?

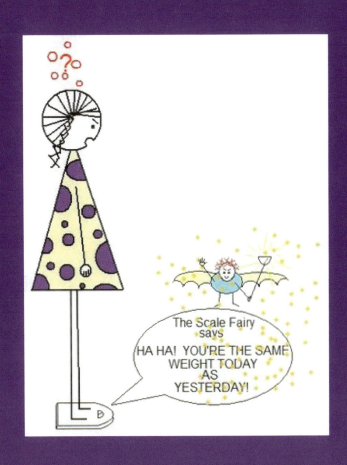

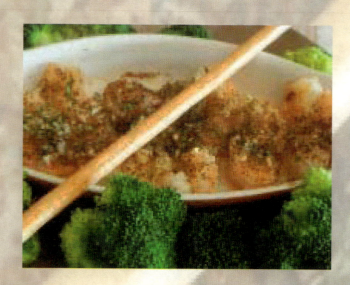

Baked Shrimp

90 calories

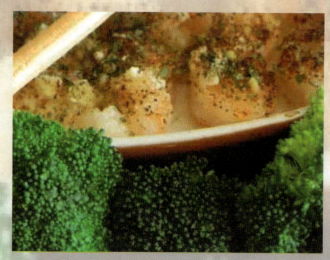

100g shrimp (90 calories)

2 cloves fresh garlic, minced

1t lime juice

a sprinkle onion powder

a sprinkle pumpkin spice

salt and pepper to taste

1t parsley

Shake ButterBuds

In a ramekin (just because it's pretty) combine everything but parsley & butter. Top shrimp with parsley and butter. Bake for approximately 8-9 minutes. I served this beside broccoli & a Parmesan grissini. It made a beautiful plate!

Going out today

So, we're planning to head out this afternoon for some yard saling and the Hood River Fly-In, which is an event where antique airplanes are displayed. It means that we won't be home this evening for dinner, though, so I've got to do a little planning.

I thought I could just go to Sub Way and order a "salad" of all tomatoes or cucumbers along with one of their broiled chicken breasts, but I've not yet done my research and want to make sure that I'd be staying on the protocol. I also considered just going to the store and purchasing some cottage cheese & veggies, take a little flavoring, a pocket knife and eat on the fly. Not so great for getting that "meal" feeling, though. Of course, that's also how I used to eat - just on the fly and what ever I could grab.

In the end I decided to do shrimp. They're easy to transport and taste good hot or cold. And shrimp, regardless of the surroundings you eat them in, are considered on some level a decadent meal. :) Obviously, that's a psychological thing. Hehehehe.

Dilly Garlic Shrimp
90 calories

100g shrimp (90 calories)

1/4t Butter Buds

1/4t garlic powder

1/2t Bragg's Liquid Aminos

1/4t dill weed

a shake or two of pepper

Place shrimp in center of 8" foil. Lay them out so they're not touching, then sprinkle butter flavor evenly over them. Then sprinkle garlic powder evenly. Then add Bragg's', trying to cover each shrimp (but don't worry about it if you don't). Over all that, spread dill weed then top with pepper. Close the foil over the shrimp, forming a little pocket and toss in the toaster oven at 350* for about 10 minutes.

"Honey" Citrus Glazed Shrimp
90 calories

100g shrimp (90 calories)
Juice of one lime, or lemon
6-10 drops orange stevia
2t Tobasco sauce
1t Ground Ginger
1/2t Celery Seed
1/4t Knox gelatin (if you want to thicken it)
Combine all ingredients except shrimp in small bowl. Add shrimp to the bowl and let marinade for an hour. Glaze will be soupy and won't look much like a glaze until it gets heated up. Center all ingredients on 8" square of foil and fold into a packet. Place in toaster oven at 350* for 10 minutes or until shrimp are done, then serve hot. I poured it all over the top of some broccoli!

This turned out to be a tasty little treat. You could sweeten it more and it'd be a kind of desert soup... But be careful if you decide to do that. Stevia has a way of dominating all other flavors.

Tonight, I'm getting ready for an all day out of town trip to Portland for cello lesson. So, I'm working to get the meatloaf and the cola chicken made up, too! I ran out of time for supper tonight, so I came up with a *really* quick shrimp recipe.

Ran-out-of-Time Asian Shrimp

90 calories

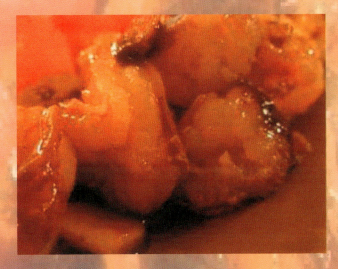

100g shrimp (90 calories)

1t Bragg's Liquid Aminos

1 garlic clove, sliced thinly

3T Walden Farms Asian dressing

In hot pan, add Bragg's and toss the shrimp in on top. Cook the shrimp fully on both sides, then turn heat off and add garlic and Asian dressing, stir so fully coated. Serve hot!

I served it up with fresh tomatoes from the garden, tossed with a little Celtic Sea Salt and served it up just as you see in the background. The tomatoes set it off nicely, adding just enough acidity to the dish to give it a nice round flavor.

I was busy working on making kids' rooms cleaner (since they don't do it). My Mom and I decided that anything that wasn't in it's proper place while they were at school today would go into a storage place until they could prove that they could keep their rooms clean.

Needless to say, lunch was selected from the ones we've already done. I know, I know. Lunch Repeater! Hahaha! Lunch today was the Chili chicken from the other day. It's a tasty and quick make.

For supper, though, I'm doing a new one. It's Shrimp Cocktail! Of course, mostly, it's the sauce that's the recipe. :) Yummy sauce, too. I served it up with yellow squash so the veggie wouldn't outshine the main course.

Shrimp Cocktail

90 calories

100g shrimp (90 calories)

1T tomato paste

1t Worcester (see Staple Sauces list)

1/2t onion powder

1/2t garlic powder

2 cloves fresh garlic, minced

1/4t celery seeds

salt & pepper to taste

1T water

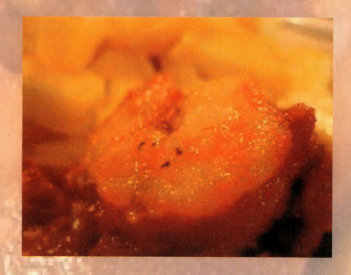

Mix everything except the shrimp in a small bowl. In ramekin, set shrimp so they don't overlap, then spoon sauce onto shrimp. Pop in the (toaster) oven 15 minutes at 325* then broil another 5 minutes. Serve it up hot!

Sushi for lunch!

You know how you have little rituals during the week, like Friday is "Sushi Day?" Well, we have one of those for when we go to Portland for music lesson. Yesterday, we didn't go to Portland, simply because it's Labor Day weekend and not a smart time to travel. But Mom and I still found ourselves craving sushi. A bad thing, considering it's not something allowed on the HCG Protocol.

Instead of just figuring we were doomed to have that craving, Mom designed a great little wanna-be sushi for us. We chose to use shrimp in ours, but crab could just as easily become the main protein here.

Wanna-be Sushi

you'll have to add up the calories

100g shrimp (90 calories) OR crab (55 calories)

1 T Plochman's stone ground mustard

1/2-1 t wasabi powder

1/2 t ground ginger

1 T Bragg's' Liquid Aminos

Onion powder to taste

Garlic powder to taste

1/2-1 t more wasabi powder

2 c Zucchini (58 calories) - you can use the allowed amount, if you like

In pan, steam zucchini until nearly done. While that's steaming, combine Plochman's, 1/2 to 1 t wasabi powder, and ginger in a small dish and set aside. Dry fry shrimp, Bragg's', onion, and garlic powders on the stove until shrimp is hot and cooked. Place shrimp in dish with mustard mixture and coat. Remove zucchini from steamer and place on plate. Place shrimp over the zucchini then, in the dish that held the mustard mixture, mix another 1/2-1 teaspoon wasabi and add 2 t water to it to make it sort of soupy, then drizzle the soupy wasabi over all of it. Tah-dah! Sushi! You can even eat it with chop sticks for the full effect. :)

Zippy Shrimp

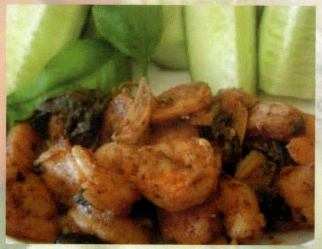

This afternoon, we're doing some zippy little shrimps. I think I'll pair it with some fresh cucumber to cool my mouth off because I plan to add more red pepper flakes and paprika to mine, but I like-a tings SPICY! In mine, I doubled a few of the ingredients, which I noted in the recipe. I tried to cool the recipe off for all you who aren't up for a spicy meal below, but my notes about how I like it are right there next to the spice that I used more of!

Zippy Shrimp
90 calories

100g jumbo shrimp (90 calories)

2T Bragg's Liquid Aminos

1/4c water

1 clove garlic, sliced

1/4t red pepper flakes (I doubled this at least for mine)

1/2t paprika (I doubled this one, too)

2T lemon juice

1 t chopped fresh basil

1/8t cinnamon

1/4t tobasco sauce

salt & pepper to taste

Heat the water and Bragg's in a skillet over medium heat; cook and stir the garlic in until the garlic is nearly translucent. Sprinkle in red pepper flakes, paprika, cinnamon, tobasco sauce, and basil. Add the shrimp and toss to coat. Pour the lemon juice over the shrimp; allow to cook until the shrimp are bright pink on the outside and the meat is no longer transparent in the center, about 1 or 2 minutes more. Reduce heat to medium-low; add the basil and toss lightly. Add your salt and pepper then serve.

A funny this morning

This morning, I started getting out my autumn and winter clothes. I put on one of my favorite shirts (the right way), but it didn't feel like it usually did. The neck was too loose.

I figured I had put it on backwards so I turned it around.

Then it really wasn't right, but this time in the shoulders. The neck felt a little tight, too. It was just not right. I checked the tag and discovered that I had turned it around so it was, indeed, backwards.

So, I turned it around yet again, front side in the front, & just had to adjust to the fact that my favorite clothes aren't going to be my favorites for much longer.

They'll be too big.

Apple Celery Soup
128 calories

1 apple (90 calories)
3c water
1T onion flakes
2c celery (38 calories)
1T beef bullion
1T chicken bullion
1/4t curry powder
1/4t paprika
1/3t lemon juice
1T milk

Peel, core, and slice apple. Cut celery into 1/2" slices. Add water, onion, bullion, curry, paprika, & lemon juice to a pan and bring to a boil. Add apple & celery to boiling broth. Allow to cook 30 minutes. Add milk at the last moment, stir it up, then serve hot!

Tonight, I'm having steak and coleslaw. It took a little adjusting to get this recipe right but it came out wonderfully in the end. I did use the optional milk for the first time ever and that was also a good choice.

The recipe makes just enough for two cups of cabbage, but you can certainly add some water to the coleslaw dressing and make it stretch if you're having more cabbage!

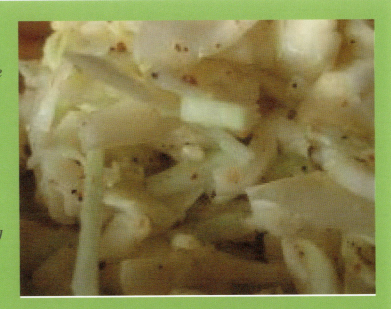

Coleslaw
35 calories

2c cabbage (35 calories)
1/2t Plochman's Natural Stone Ground mustard
1/2t lemon juice
shake of celery seeds
2-3 drops stevia
shake of onion powder
salt
pepper
1T milk

Slice up cabbage real fine and set in a bowl to refrigerate. Mix all other ingredients in small bowl and drizzle over the cabbage. Stir the cabbage so the dressing coats it completely. Return to the frig for at least an hour before serving.

Liquid Sunshine Soup
31 calories

Allowed amount yellow squash (1c=31 calories)
juice of one lemon
2 drops Stevia
Veggie broth (1 1/2 cups or so)
1t onion powder
1/2t cumin
1/2t coriander
1t cinnamon
3/4t powdered ginger
1/2t powdered mustard
cayenne to taste
salt & pepper to taste

Roast the squash by cutting in half, removing seeds and stringy membrane (you can add this to the soup if you don't mind the "guts," but definitely do this step, as it adds to the lovely flavor), place cut side down on baking sheet, pierce skin with a fork a few times, cook at 350 for 40 minutes or until soft.

Scoop squash flesh away from skin and puree with lemon juice. Add all ingredients in with the broth. Simmer gently until flavors are mixed.

Waldorf Salad
79 calories

1/2 apple, chopped, leaving peel on (40 calories)
1 bunch celery hearts, sliced thin (39 calories)
Leave the peel on the apple, but not the little sticker. :) Salt apples and toss. Add celery and toss with apples. Toss with Vinnegrape Dressing (below) and serve.

Vinnegrape Dressing

2T Walden Farms Grape jelly
1 1/2T Marukan Light & Mild rice vinegar
6 whole allspice
10 anise seeds
1 1/2t water
Bring dressing just to a full rolling boil, then remove from heat. Don't eat the allspice!

Raspberry Picking

Yesterday, when we went for our outing, we headed for some of the local farms to get some *really* fresh fruit. It actually started as an outing for the kids to go enjoy the pumpkin patch and the corn maze. Both of those things turned out to be "soooo boring" and we swiftly looked for other things to do.

So, off to some of the farms to see if we could find some pony rides or something like that. What we found were autumn raspberries, honey crisp apples, the last of the peaches for the season, and we picked up some pears off the ground after the pickers had already picked off the trees. Mom's making peach/pineapple jam, pear butter, and apple butter and canning (why do they call it canning when you're using jars?) them for use during the winter. We also grabbed up some fresh tomatoes to stew and freeze for later in the winter. There's nothing like the taste of fresh picked, even if it comes out of the freezer.

Anyway, while we were picking raspberries, I figured that this was just going to be my fruit for the afternoon. I think I ate 3x the amount of raspberries I was allowed, but YUMMY!! Pick, pick, pick, eat, eat, pick, pick, pick, eat, eat, pick...

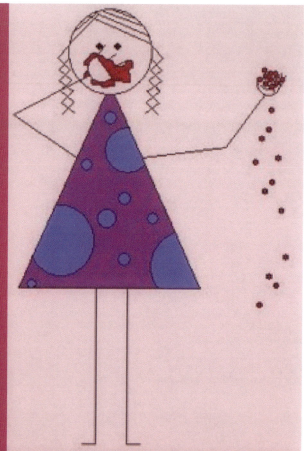

So, it's time to figure out some ways to make eating while on this protocol a little more portable. It's all well and good if you can just stay home and make all your meals. It's not so cool for anyone who needs to eat *gasp* at work or while out on vacation!

I'll start with desert, just because it's an easy place to start.

Apple Chips

1 apple, cored
Juice of one lemon
10 drops cinnamon stevia

Preheat oven to 300°F. Cut apples as thinly as possible, crosswise into circles. Set aside. Mix lemon juice and stevia together, then brush onto one side of each apple slice. Place sweetened side down on a baking sheet covered with parchment paper. Bake until golden brown, about 12 minutes.

Store in an airtight container in a cool dry place. Do not refrigerate or they become soft and sticky.

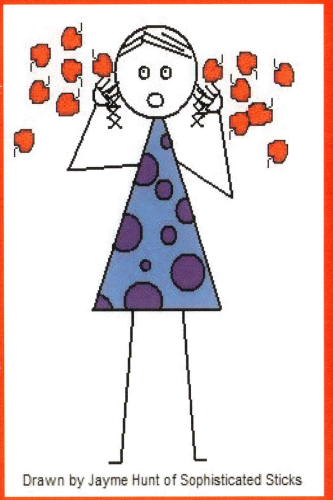

Drawn by Jayme Hunt of Sophisticated Sticks

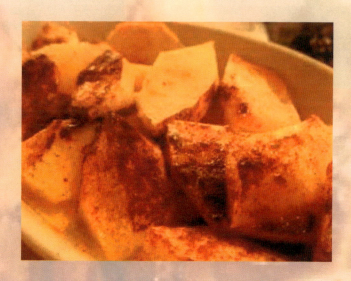

Sweet Toffee Apple
80 calories

1 gala apple (80 calories)

1t butter buds

16 drops Toffee Stevia

1/2t cinnamon

1/4t nutmeg

dash salt

1T milk

Core and cut apple into quarters, then slice them about 1" thick. Put apple in ramekin. Sprinkle with butter, toffee stevia, cinnamon, nutmeg, and salt. Pour milk over the top of all of it. Place in oven, uncovered 30 minutes at 350* then broil an additional 10 minutes.

These two recipes really help get a person through Phase Two of the Protocol. Between dark cocoa and something that tastes similar to the insides of an apple pie, you just can't stumble while staying on this protocol. Here's to Less of Us!

White Dark Cocoa
0 calories

30 drops Dark Chocolate Stevia (made by NOW Foods)
20 oz HOT water
Mix the two and drink up - it's a freebie!

Zippy Baked Cinnamon Apple
80 calories

1 medium Gala apple (80 calories)
1/4t cinnamon
1/4t nutmeg
1/8t chili powder
1/2t cloves (if you like)
6-10 drops Stevia (or Vanilla Stevia)
Cut apple (I used the Gala apples because they're a little more tart and juicy than other apples right now, at the beginning of September) in half and core so there's no seeds and you have a little hole in the middle. Sprinkle the seasonings over the top of the apple halves, then add the Stevia, one drop at a time until you think it's going to be sweet enough. Bake in the toaster oven (yah, it's still summer here and we use this more often than the big oven cuz it doesn't heat the whole house up) at 350* for 30 to 45 minutes.

This afternoon's treat was just that - a real treat! See how beautiful it was? It was so delightful, in fact, that I had trouble naming this dish. Orange Crème de Licious? Orange Crème de Wonderful? Orange Crème de Lovely?

Orange Crème de Licious

60 calories

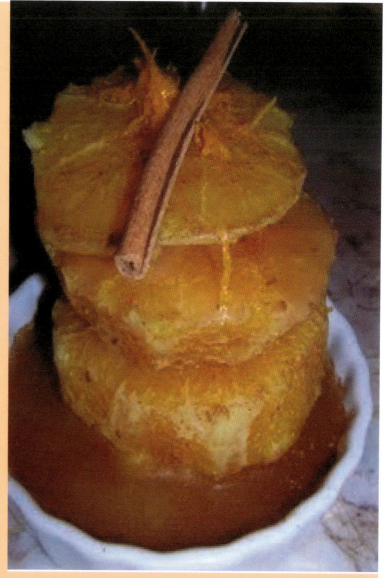

1 Orange (60 calories)
4 cinnamon sticks
8 whole allspice
8 whole cloves
1 can Ginger Ale Zevia
2 drops vanilla creme stevia
1T milk

Peel orange. Get as much of the white off as you can. Slice into four rounds. Break four 4" cinnamon sticks into large pieces, 8 whole allspice also broken into large pieces - so they're not completely pulverized, but they're open. To that, add 8 whole cloves. Pour them into a coffee filter (or gauze or muslin), and form a spice envelope.

Put spice envelope into a deep bowl. Lay orange rounds over that. Cover all that with Zevia Ginger Ale. Weight it down with another bowl so the spices and oranges stay completely covered by the Zevia.

Let stand overnight to mull.

When it's done mulling, carefully pick out your orange slices. If you can get the spices out without them leaking, that's great, otherwise you'll have to strain the spices out of the Zevia. To the spiced ginger ale, add stevia, put on stove and reduce some. Add ground ginger (to taste), reduce more, then pour over the orange slices.

Garnish with a whole cinnamon stick or two for a real show stopper!

Chef's Notes: For pretty pictures, I strained out the "dregs" of spices from the reduction. It's not strictly necessary, but does make it look better!

We've recently discovered the jellies that Walden Farms makes. Raspberry is the jelly of choice these days, but the grape is still waiting in the wings. We also want to do something with the apricot jelly, but I'm not sure what to do with it yet. Soon!

Raspberry Apple

90 calories

apple (90 calories)
1t Walden Farms Raspberry jelly
1t cinnamon
1/2t nutmeg
1/2t butter buds
1T milk
1pkg stevia

Cut up apple into bite sized pieces and place in ramekin. In small bowl, mix jelly, cinnamon, nutmeg, butter buds, and milk, then drizzle over apples. Sprinkle stevia over all that, cover with foil. Place in oven at 350* for 30 minutes.

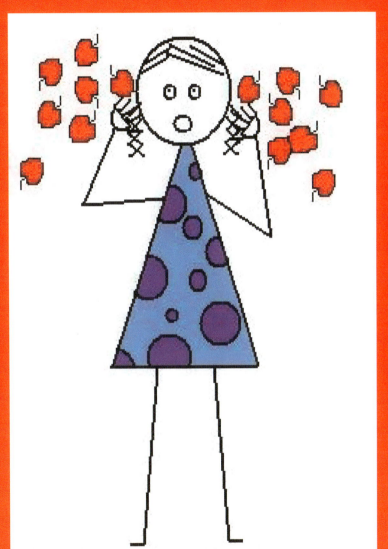

Tonight, we've put a little bit of a twist on an old friend. The Baked Cinnamon Apple is delicious, but even the best things in life get tedious after a while. It's time for a new take on that old favorite. I actually have a two-fer for you this evening, depending on your choice of tart or sweet. The addition of the lemon to the one recipe turned out a very different taste - delicious and like a sweet tart candy. The other was very toffee and just as delicious as the first.

The milk gives it just enough creaminess that you feel really spoiled and I honestly couldn't tell you which I like better! I'm sure you'll love both, too.

Tart Toffee Apple

80 calories

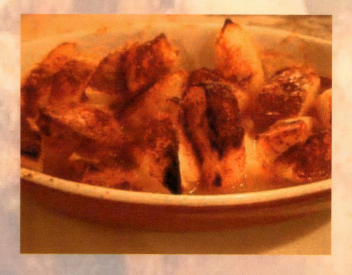

1 gala apple (80 calories)

1t lemon juice

1t butter buds

16 drops Toffee Stevia

1/2t cinnamon

1/4t nutmeg

dash salt

1T milk

Core and cut apple into quarters, then slice them about 1" thick. Add slices to a bowl and pour lemon juice over the top of it. Let sit for at least 1/2 hour. Put apple in ramekin. Sprinkle with butter, toffee stevia, cinnamon, nutmeg, and salt. Pour milk over the top of all of it. Place in oven, uncovered 30 minutes at 350* then broil an additional 10 minutes.

Yogurt

1c cottage cheese
2pkg stevia
1t agar agar
2T milk
1t vanilla
2 grissini sticks
Blend all ingredients until really smooth. Let it blend for 5-7 minutes. Makes a double batch, so be sure to eat only half! To serve, you could add your fruit to the bottom of the bowl and top with this yogurt. It makes a quick on the go type meal.

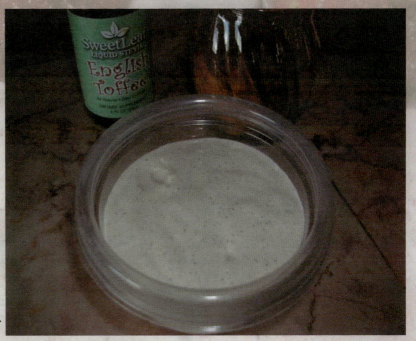

Lemon Christilicious Yogurt

1/2 Yogurt Recipe
Juice of one lemon
2 grissini sticks
Blend all ingredients until really smooth. Let it blend for 5-7 minutes.

Cinnamon Yogurt

1/2 Yogurt Recipe
1/2t cinnamon
1/4t nutmeg
Blend all ingredients until really smooth. Let it blend for 5-7 minutes.

Lime Yogurt

1/2 Yogurt Recipe
Juice of one lime
2 grissini sticks
Blend all ingredients until really smooth. Let it blend for 5-7 minutes.

Raspberry Cheesecake

1 Cinnamon Yogurt Recipe
Allowed amount raspberries
12 drops berry stevia
Toss raspberries with 12 drops berry stevia. Put berries in ramekin, cover with yogurt Chill 1 hour.

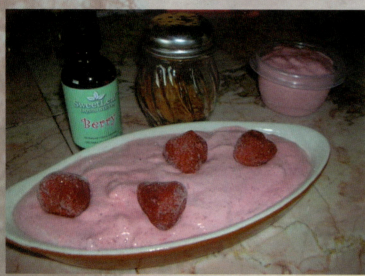

Chilled Strawberry Pudding

1 Cinnamon Yogurt Recipe
2c strawberry
12 drops berry stevia
Mix all ingredients in blender and blend for 5-7 minutes, making sure the berries get blended up, too. Pour into ramekin and chill at least one hour.

Chilled Apple Pudding

1 Cinnamon Yogurt Recipe
1 medium apple
12 drops toffee stevia
Slice apple into thin slices and bake until done (about 45 minutes at 350*). Mix all ingredients in blender and blend for 5-7 minutes, making sure the apples get blended up, too. Pour into ramekin and chill at least one hour. Drizzle Walden Farms Caramel Sauce on top, if you'd like!

Orange Jaymeus

1/2 Yogurt recipe
Juice of an orange
12-15 drops french vanilla stevia
6 ice cubes
Juice the orange really well, so there's only juice. Add to blender, along with remaining ingredients until really smooth. Let it blend for 1-2 minutes. Garnish with a slice of orange on the rim of the glass for a very pretty desert.

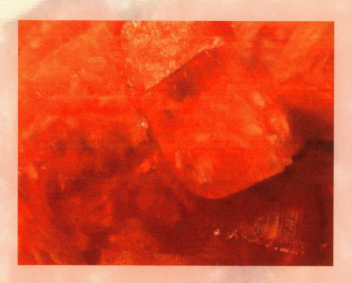

Serious big YUMMMMMMYY!! This recipe is thicker than regular Jello so it would stand well for travel and such. I'm not sure you should leave it out of the frig all day long, but if you put it into an insulated lunch bag with a cold pack, this should hold up really well.

Raspberry Jello

52 calories per serving - makes 2 servings

1c raspberries (64 calories)
1/2c water
33 drops stevia
1/2c Natural Twist Zevia (Lemon Lime)
2 envelopes Knox Gelatin (40 calories)
Mash raspberries and add water and stevia. Bring this just to a boil. In separate bowl, pour Zevia in, add gelatin and let sit 1 minute. Add fruit and stevia mix to gelatin mixture and stir 5 minutes. Pour into pie dish or ramekins or other container. (Note: This recipe is **<u>doubled</u>** so I could pour it into an 8x10 pan.) Refrigerate at least 3 hours and serve!

Of note, when making this, I left the seeds *in* the dish. Where I considered straining them out, I was afraid that I'd lose the fiber from the whole berry, which would be in the raspberry if I were just to eat it whole. To stick to the protocol, that's why I made it and left the berry seeds in.

Raspberry Sorbet

Tonight, we present something that happened a little by accident. A happy accident to be sure, but an accident none the less. It was supposed to be a variation on a recipe shared by a friend, but all I had was frozen berries, so we had to do some alterations to make the blender blend!

What we did is below - it's a great desert recipe that you ought to keep in your back pocket while in Phase Two of the HCG Protocol. :)

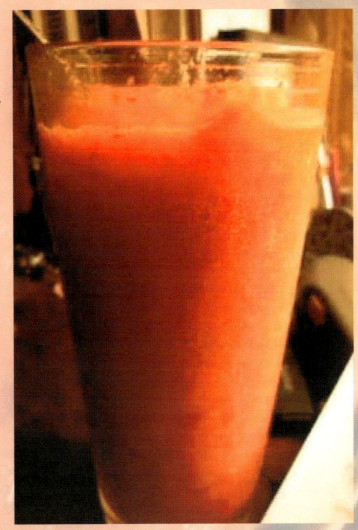

Raspberry Sorbet

32 calories

1/2c frozen raspberries (32 calories)

15 drops Berry stevia

1/2 can Orange Zevia

1/4c water

Blend the ingredients together and enjoy with a spoon! YUMMY!

Egg Day!

Today, I've decided to try something that's not in the Pounds and Inches (P&I) book. I've read, on a forum I frequent, about a Phase 2 Egg Day. It takes the place of the Apple Day and is ONLY used for breaking a stall. The gist of it is that you eat 6 WHOLE eggs through out the day - 3 for lunch, 3 for dinner.

I think it's supposed to simulate the loading days, as the yolks have quite a bit of fat in them - 14g each yolk, in fact. I did break my last stall of 13 days, with a QXCI session from Tami (daniels at gorge dot net), where I get my hCG.

(Aside: She sells all the vitamins you should be taking, including the hCG, too!)

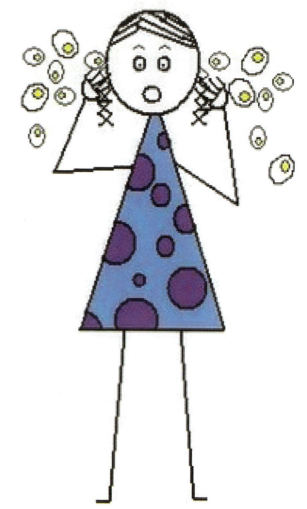

Drawn by Jayme Hunt of Sophisticated Sticks

QXCI is kind of expensive, though, at $150 per 2 hour session and I can't use that every time I'm at a stall. Two days after the QXCI, I released 4 pounds. Since then, Monday, I've been at the same 305.4# day in and day out. WHAT is my body doing?? It should be just melting the fat away - I've been SO good while following this protocol.

So, for educational purposes – and you should note that this is not part of the original P&I Protocol – here's what I'm doing today:

> *The egg day is used in place of an apple day to break a stall/plateau ONLY.*
>
> *Eat six eggs in a single day, for a total of 447 calories.**
>
> *I'm never hungry when I do an egg day and I'm usually down at least one pound the following morning.*

Another person warns, though:

> *As a cautionary tale...do not abuse this! I did abuse this during my last round and now that I'm on Phase 3 my beloved egg days won't work anymore. The first time I used it I was going to be traveling and stuck in a hospital all day so it was more of a convenience thing, but then I did it I think 2 more times just to try to get down to a certain weight, and a little because I'm lazy too and can buy bags of peeled cooked hard boiled eggs at my Trader Joe's and I get really sick of meat by the end of Phase 2.**

*Posts found on the happilythinnerafter.com forums.

Final Notes

Time/Labor Savers for Phase 2

Jill, on the Yahoo forum, posted this message that I thought we should all be thinking about. Why reinvent the wheel, after all? She asks and answers her own question with suggestions of her own:

What are your favorite time or labor savers on this diet?

- For both my rounds of HCG/VLCDieting, I bought enough meat for all my meals for the full course in one trip. I went home and immediately weighed out the portions and put them into individual baggies and froze them.

- My proteins for this round are cube steak, sirloin tips, ground veal (mixed with fresh garlic, parsley, sage, rosemary, and thyme), veal scaloppini, chicken breast, shrimp, tilapia, and mahi-mahi.

- Every day at lunch, I move two protein servings from the freezer to the fridge so they are thawed for the following day's lunch/dinner.

- Bought quite a few grapefruit, oranges, lemons, and apples because they last a pretty long time in the fridge.

- That leaves a quick weekly trip for fresh vegetables and strawberries. I have plenty of spices, apple cider vinegar, and sea salt on hand. I also have excellent beef and chicken stock made by the Amish farmers I get most of my food from.

- When I am making a meal, while the protein and veggies cook I think about what I'll have for the next meal, and try to do any prep, such as marinate the meat in a mix of interesting spices and maybe vinegar, or chop the vegetables. Some large vegetables, for example a head of cabbage, I chop up and put in 2c portions in the fridge to eat over several days. Also, a few vegetables are just fine warmed up...I will typically cook a large amount of chard to have at 2-4 meals, for example.

- I'm not as big on reheating meat so I almost always cook that fresh for each meal. I cook the protein (except for shrimp) on a small George Foreman grill; pretty much anything is cooked in 3 minutes. I sprinkle various herbs on the meat before I cook it. Sometimes I put on the herbs the night before to let them marinate. (The shrimp I cook in a saucepan with equal parts water and ACV, and Old Bay seasoning. I eat it with a homemade cocktail sauce of organic no sugar added ketchup and a generous dollop of prepared horseradish.)

- I make a quantity of salad dressing out of crushed garlic mashed into a paste with Celtic sea salt, equal parts fresh lemon juice and red wine vinegar, and a generous dollop of dijon mustard.

- This round, based on my experience from last round, I bought several heads of garlic. Today when I was cooking my meal, I peeled all the cloves from one head and put them in the fridge. I like to use a lot of garlic, but peeling cloves is a drag, so I did a bunch at once. Last time I got a large container of peeled garlic cloves, but this time I wanted to use organic and the two organic markets nearest me didn't sell garlic that way. If you want to use a container like that, if you cook only for yourself you might find some of them spoil before you finish them. I would vacuum pack half the cloves next time if I bought a container. (Or you could freeze half.)

- For my first round I had already gradually switched to decaffeinated coffee. This round I am going without coffee altogether, wondering if that little bit of caffeine in the decaf is enough to slow down my weight loss and healing. I am drinking water with lemon, sea salt, and ACV; hot and iced herbal teas; WuLong tea as recommended by Trudeau (that might have some caffeine in it, I am not sure yet); and Dandy Blend, a coffee substitute made of ground dandelion roots, chicory, and I think beet roots (jar isn't in front of me at the moment). It's pretty good. I also use that in cold raw milk when I am drinking milk...it's delicious, naturally sweet...helps me keep drinking my raw milk even when it's just beginning to naturally sour (like yogurt, as opposed to pasteurized milk, which just spoils). The Dandy Blend masks the sour taste pretty well and unlike chocolate powder it's naturally sweet and doesn't have caffeine. It has kind of a chocolate/carob/coffee flavor.

Now, we'll add to that list with a few more shortcuts:
- We, bought the meat for a week or more and froze it, too. We did it a little differently than Jill suggested, though. We used ziplock sandwich/snack baggies and bagged each serving in a single bag. Then we took a gallon freezer ziplock bag, labeled it with a Sharpie as to the kind of meat it contained, then all the little bags went into the one big bag and we didn't have to label each individual baggie.
- Chop up your apples in either quarters or slices and freeze them for your desserts. They cook just as fast and are easier to deal with.
- Make up a lot of the Staple Sauces from this book as well as the salad dressing of your choice (We just purchased the Walden Farms dressings and used those). Get at least a dozen 1 ounce glass bottles. Fill 2 bottles with each of the Staple Sauces, and 2 bottles with your choices of dressing(s) so you can just grab and go.
- Cook up at least 2 different meats, going pretty bland on the seasonings, and freeze them. This way if you get into a time crunch, you can just grab one of those, your salad dressing bottle, and head out. You can stop at a restaurant and get a lettuce only salad, add your meat and dressing, and you're set for a quick satisfying meal.

Resources

Bragg's Products (Amino Acids & Apple Cider Vinegar)
    http://www.bragg.com
    Bragg Live Foods, Inc.
    Box 7, Santa Barbara, CA 93102
    info@bragg.com
    Phone 800.446.1990
    Fax 805.968.1001

Walden Farms
    http://www.waldenfarms.com
    Phone 800.229.1706

Zevia
    http://www.zevia.com
    Zevia LLC
    zevia@zevia.com
    500 Union Street, Suite 1025, Seattle, WA 98101
    Phone 800.230.2221

Homeopathic HCG Drops
    Daniel's Health LLC
    1411 13th St, Hood River, OR 97031
    Phone: 541.386.7328
    daniels@gorge.net

SweetLeaf Stevia
    http://www.sweetleaf.com
    Wisdom Natural Brands™ - Makers of SweetLeaf Sweetener®
    info@wisdomnaturalbrands.com
    1203 W. San Pedro St, Gilbert, AZ 85233
    Phone 800.899.9908

NOW Foods Stevia
    NOW Foods
    395 S. Glen Ellyn Road, Bloomingdale, IL 60108
    Phone 888.669.3663

Finding the best price on the products that help you stay on Phase II isn't hard if you utilize a free tool we used during Phase II:

http://www.google.com/products
Just enter the name of the product you're looking for and use the drop down menu to organize by price, low to high. It's a bit difficult to wade through the irrelevant stuff, but we found that http://www.allstarhealth.com generally had the lowest prices on Stevia.

If you find that you need some help and support, we found that Jason Hill at http://www.pounds-and-inches.com offers FREE consulting and support! You can email him at info@pounds-and-inches.com. In our experience, he gets back to you with an answer within, at most, half an hour!

The best (and more expensive) hand cream we found is Great Scott Medicated Skin Cream:
    http://www.greatscottskincream.com
    elizabeth@greatscottskincream.com
    Phone 866.299.9379

The least expensive and readily available hand creme is Corn Husker's Lotion. You can find this in just about any grocery or drug store. It's generally under $5.00.

Finally, our blog & websites will continue to be updated as we go through more rounds of HCG. We also have plans to release a few more books!
    http://www.lessofmehcg.com
    http://www.madeinboyd.com
    Made In Boyd, LLC
    lessofmehcg@gmail.com
    66370 Boyd Loop Rd, Boyd, OR 97021

Here's to Less of Me & YOU!

About the Authors

Christine & Jayme are mother and daughter who live in Boyd, OR with a large family of both people and animals.

Christine enjoys reading, landscaping, gardening, woodworking, cooking, sewing, ironing, building tree houses, and setting up rope swings for her grandchildren. She really doesn't like cobwebs, spiders in the house, dog nose prints on the car windows, and putting away dishes or laundry.

Jayme enjoys spending time with her dogs, playing cello, Animal Communication, Quantum Touch, Quantum Jumping, Astronomy (the night sky at Boyd is perfect for star viewing!), mastering new things, and playing Scrabble. She really doesn't like eating lima beans, brussel sprouts, or mushrooms and she really hates doing dishes. Jayme plans to go through the HCG Protocol at least twice more in 2010.

This is Jayme after the first round of HCG:

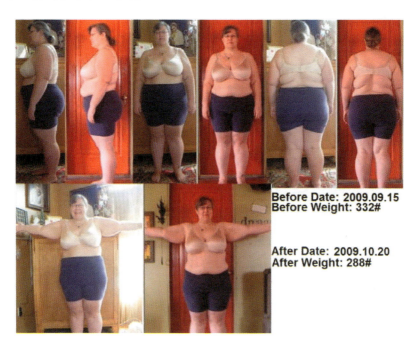

Before Date: 2009.09.15
Before Weight: 332#

After Date: 2009.10.20
After Weight: 288#

As of the publish date of this book, Jayme is maintaining the weight of 287 pounds and is in Phase Four.

Made in the USA
Lexington, KY
05 July 2010